What's Going on in There??

Let's Learn About Epilepsy

Spike and the Gang Series: Book 2

By: Leslie Pedreira, APRN

This book series is dedicated to all the amazing patients I have had the privilege of caring for through the years! Your courage and strength inspired me to write these books!

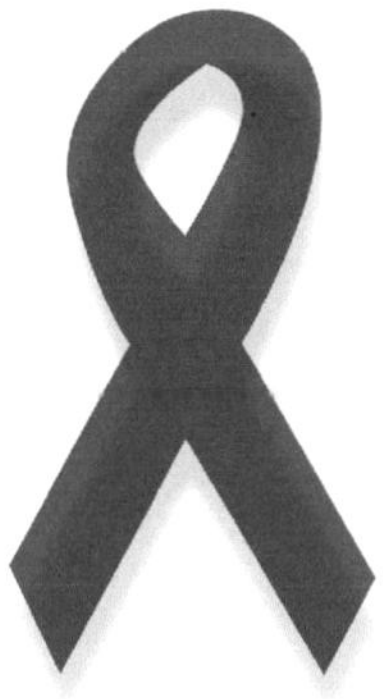

Remember us??

In case you forgot, my name is Spike. This is my friend Sharpie and my cousin Polly.

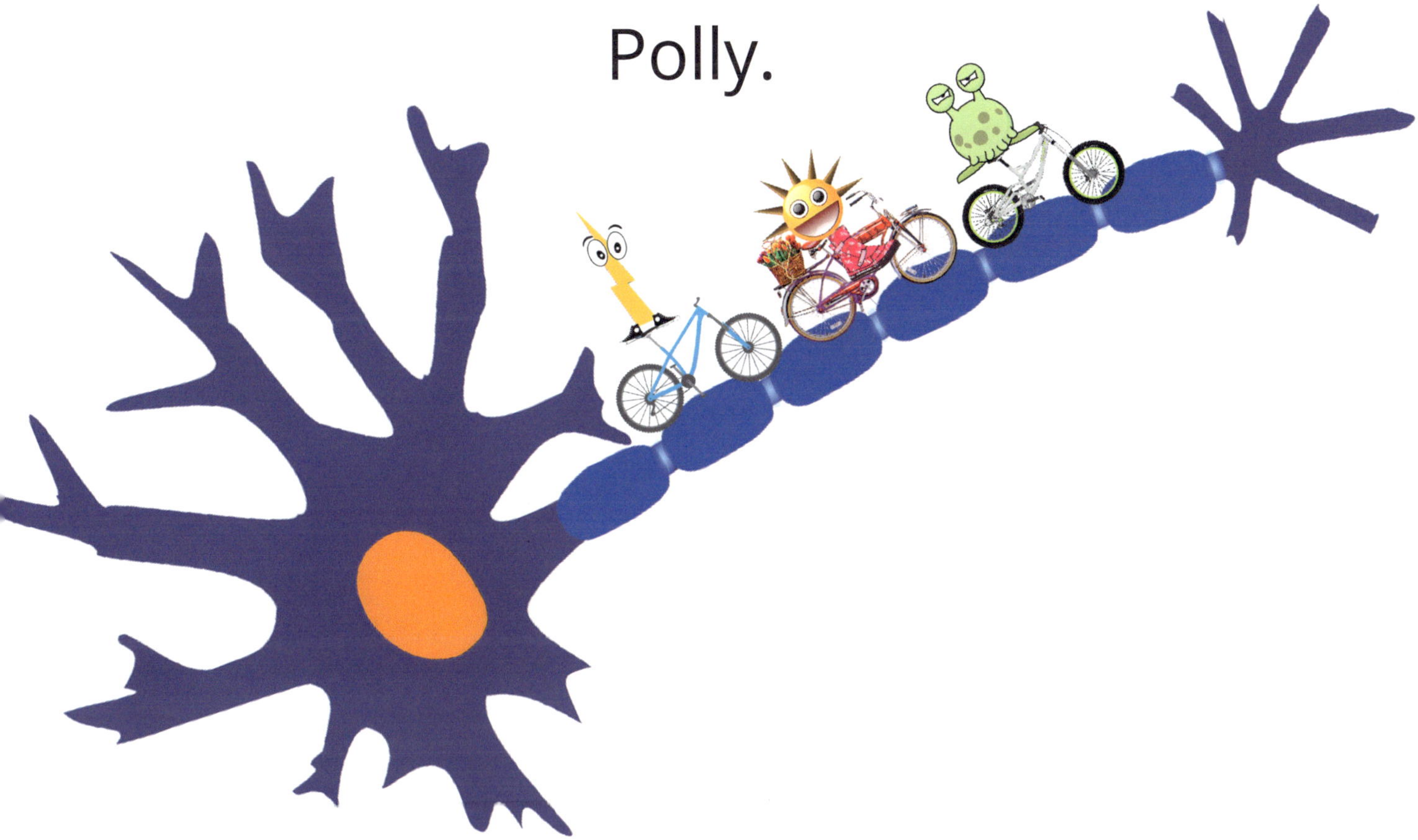

Today we are going to tell you a little bit about each of us!

Since I am the star of the show, I will go first!

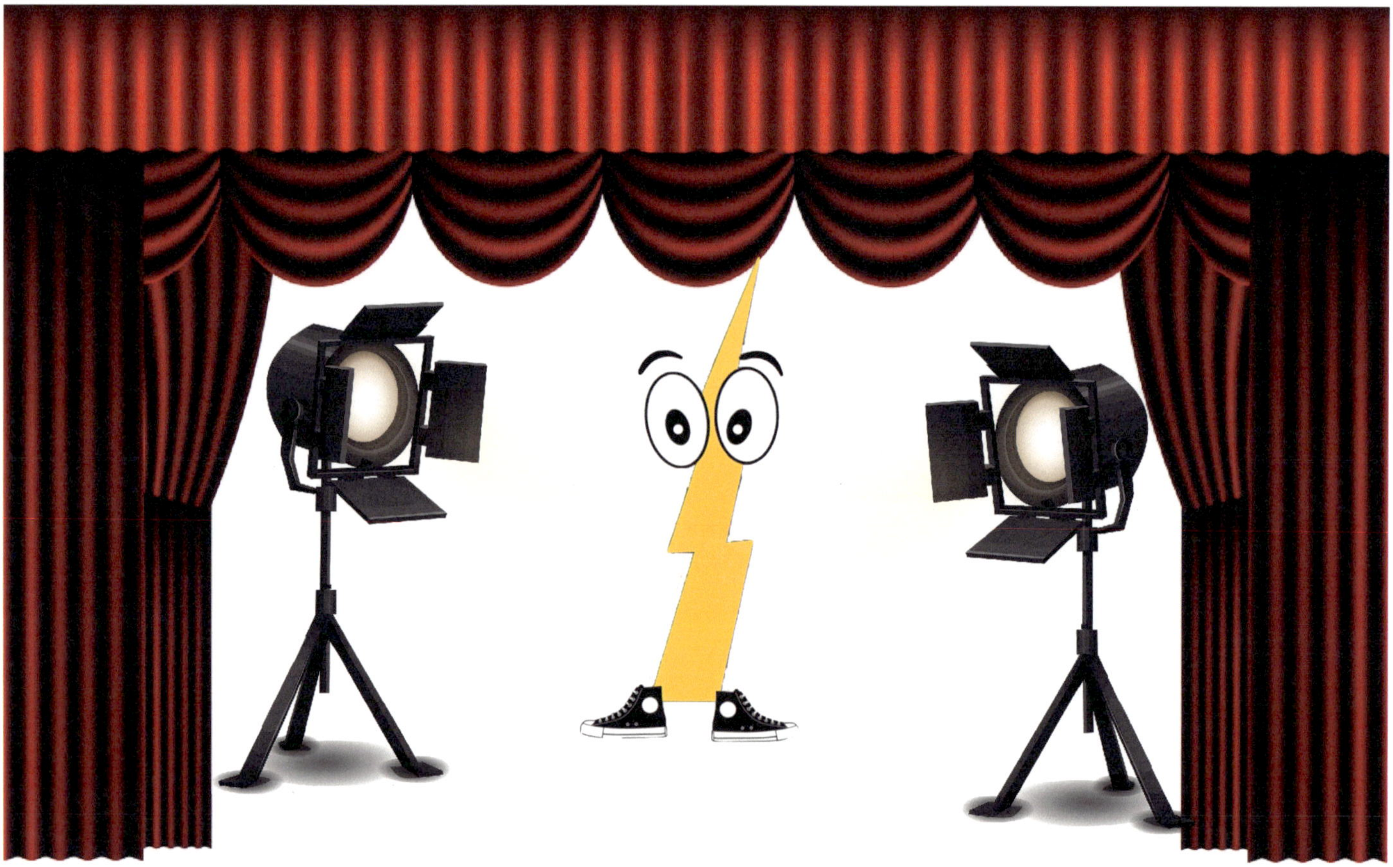

I am a Spike. I am tall, strong and I can make you have a seizure when I am in a bad mood.

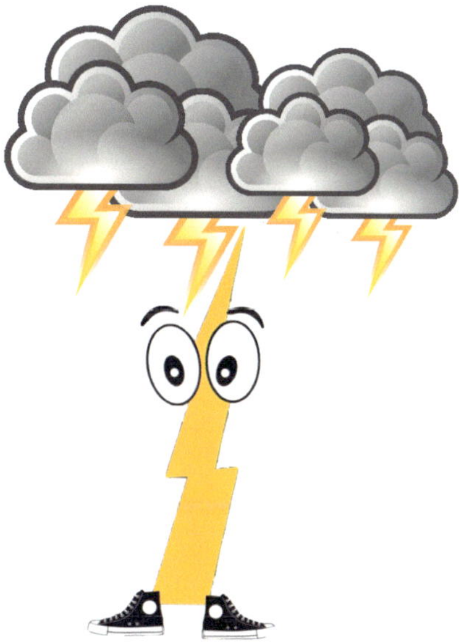

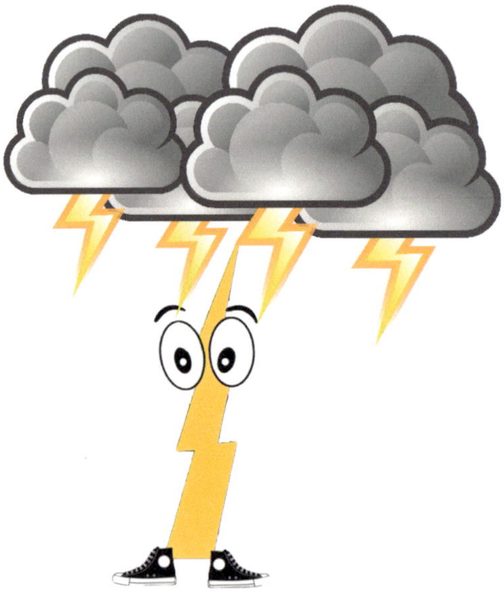

HOW DO I DO IT??

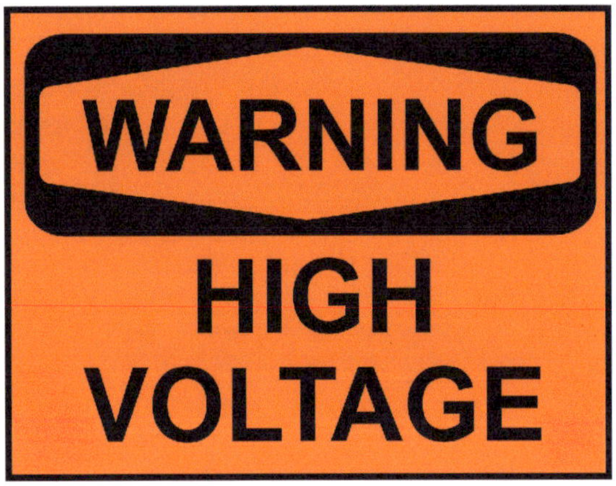

When I get mad, I can change the way your brain works. When I get really, really mad I can send my electrical spikes really fast across your brain over and over again. This can cause you to have a seizure.

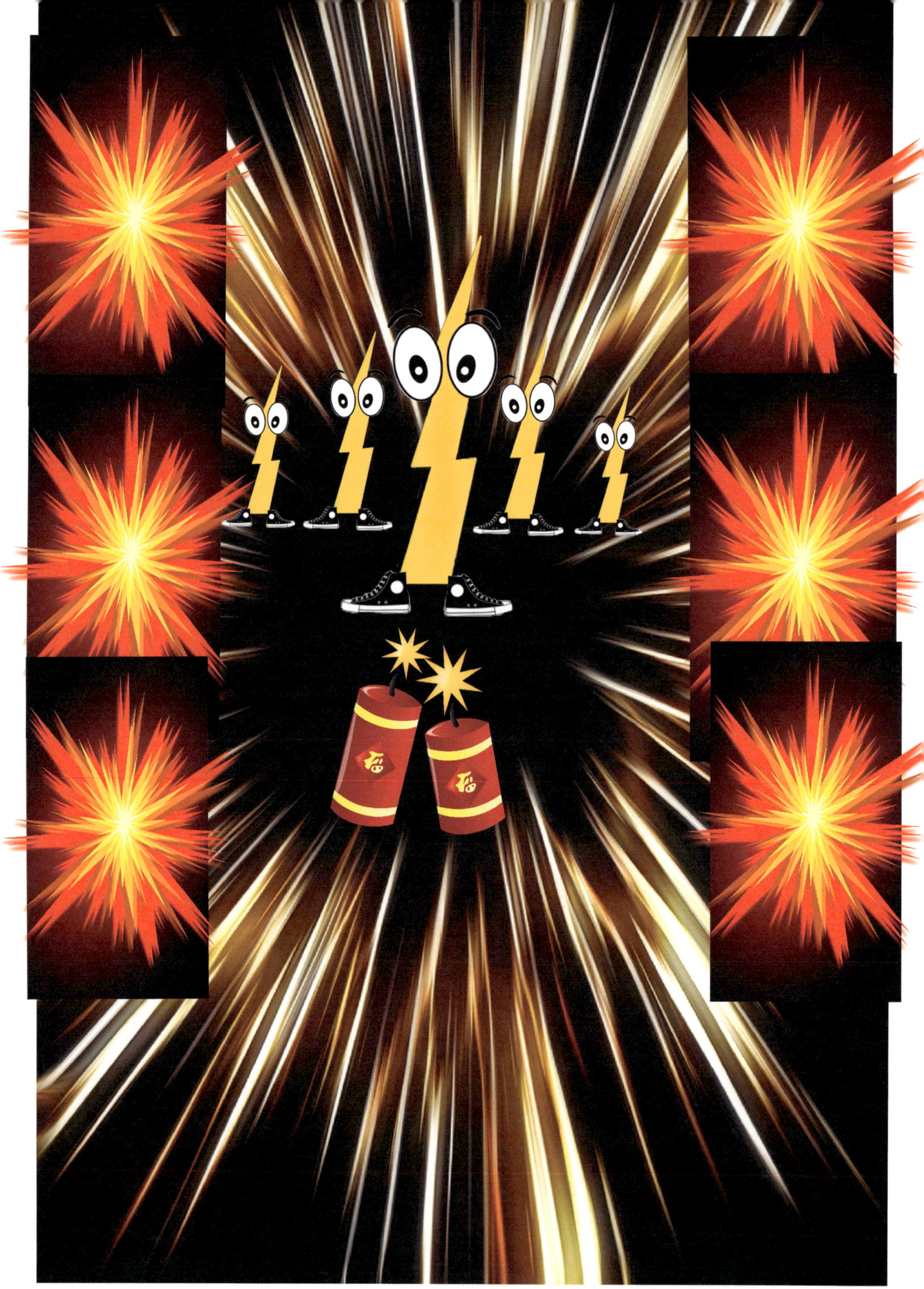

I can send my spikes across your entire brain at one time over and over again really really fast causing a generalized (jen-er-uh-lized) seizure.

This type of seizure may make you fall and shake.

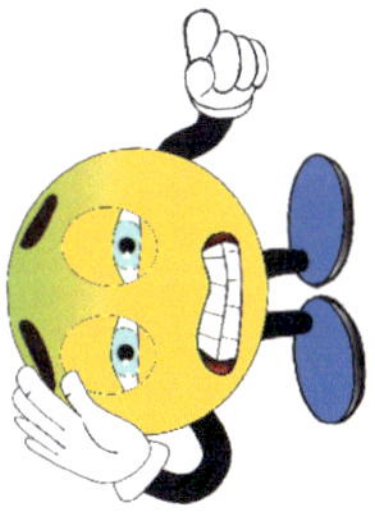

Your eyes may roll back and your muscles may hurt. You may bite down really hard on your tongue. You may even pee, poop or throw up (ewww did I really just say that?). Let's move on...

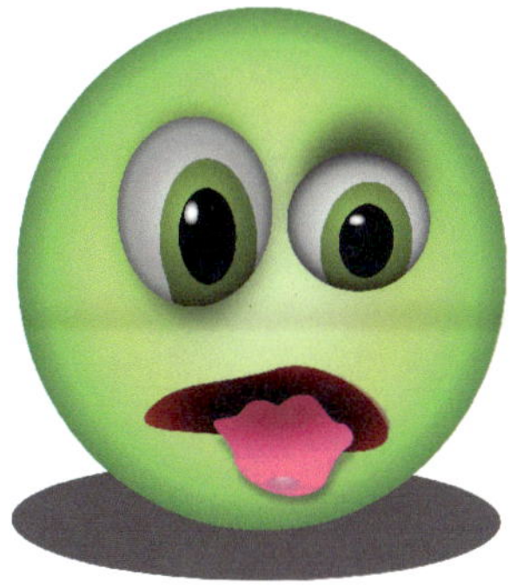

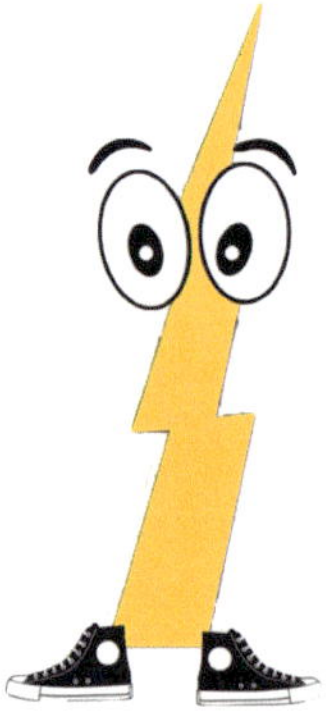

You may not feel well once it is over.

You may want to sleep and you may have a headache. This is normal. Usually, you will not remember what happened.

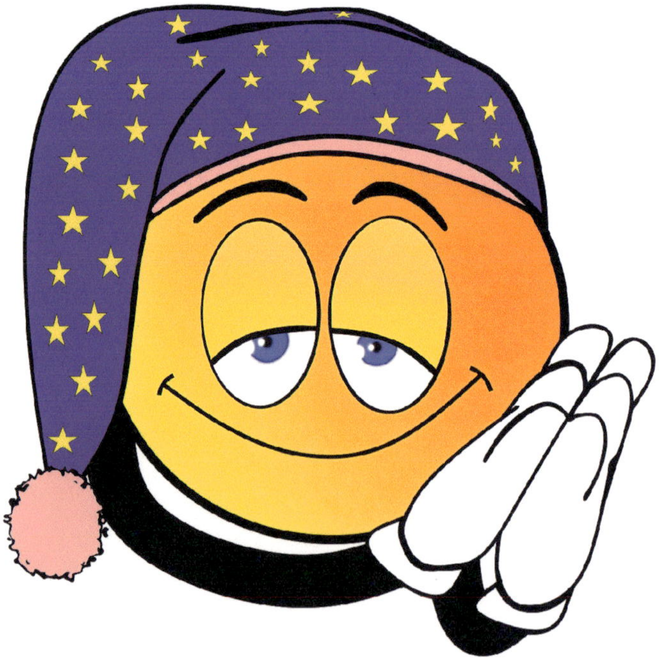

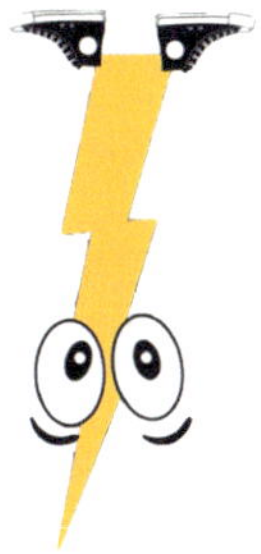

I can send my electrical spikes over just one area of your brain if I want to. This type of seizure can look different depending on where I am living.

It may make one side of your face or mouth twitch or move funny

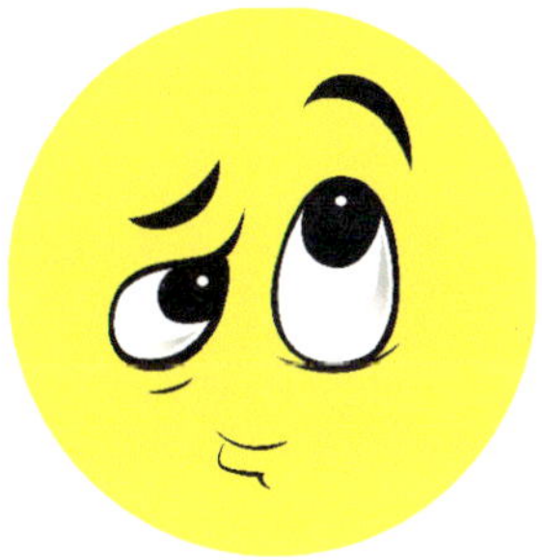

you may be able to hear but not talk

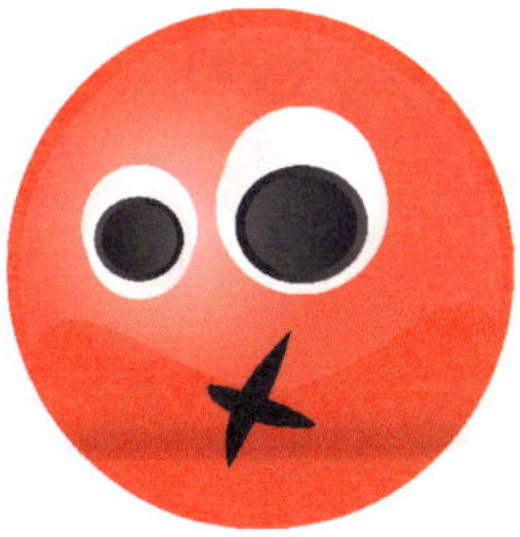

you may be able to talk and hear, but when you talk it does not come out right

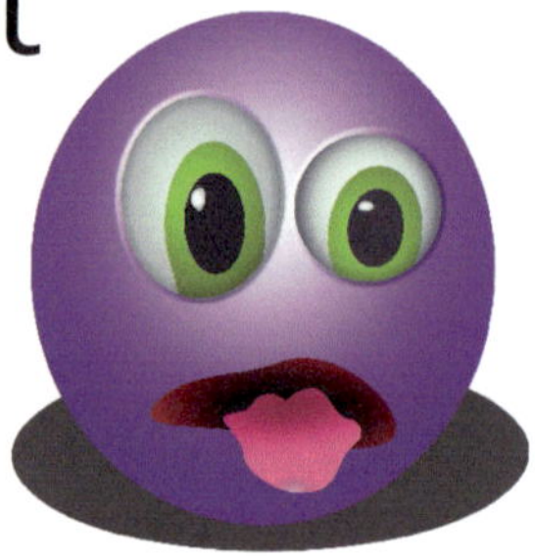

you may be confused or dizzy

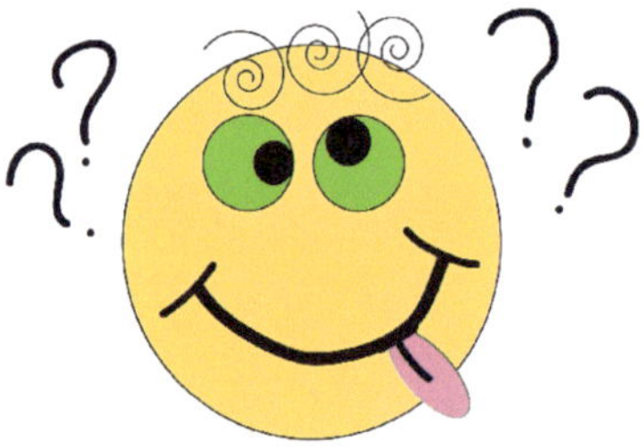

Half of your body may do some wierd stuff. Your arm or leg may get sore or stiff and you can't stop it.

do not worry--this is normal

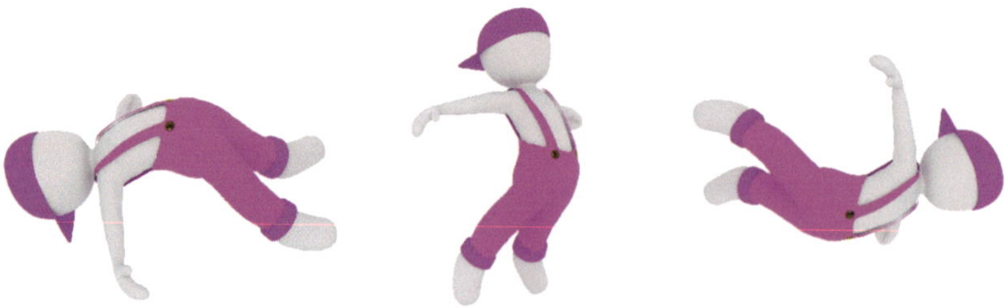

Focal (foe-cull) seizures can also make you throw up or have a headache. You may not know who mommy and daddy are for a few minutes. Do not worry.

You are safe and they will take care of you

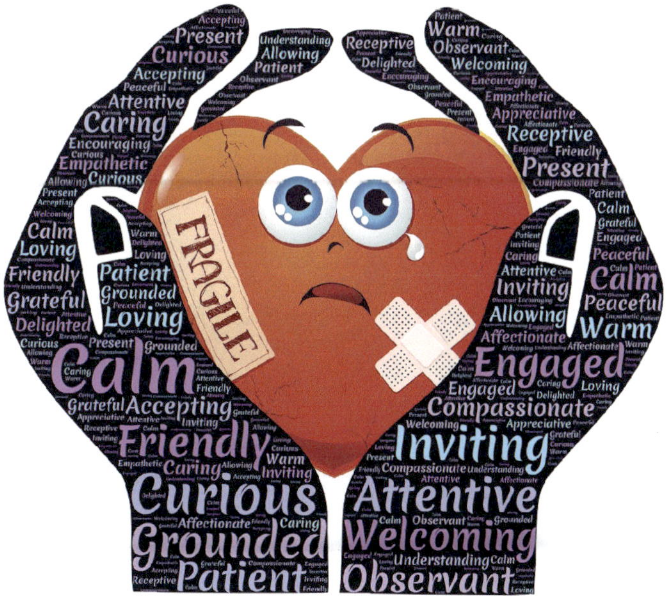

Some people get warnings before they have seizures. This is called an Aura.

Auras may happen with focal (foe-cull) seizures.

Some people notice:

seeing colors, lines, spots or objects

hearing things

funny smells

feelings of deja-vu (that's a big word that means you feel you have already been somewhere before)

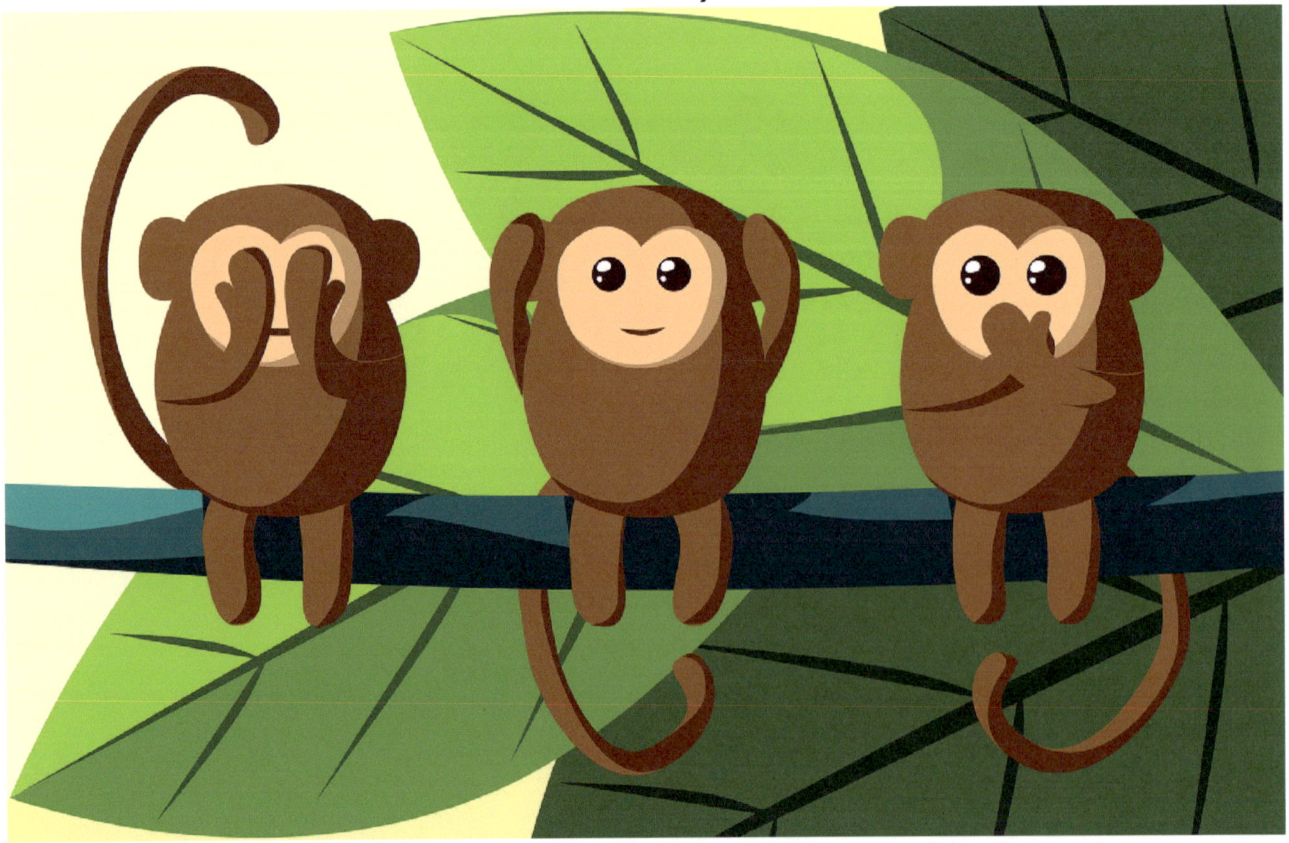

Now you know about me and what I can do

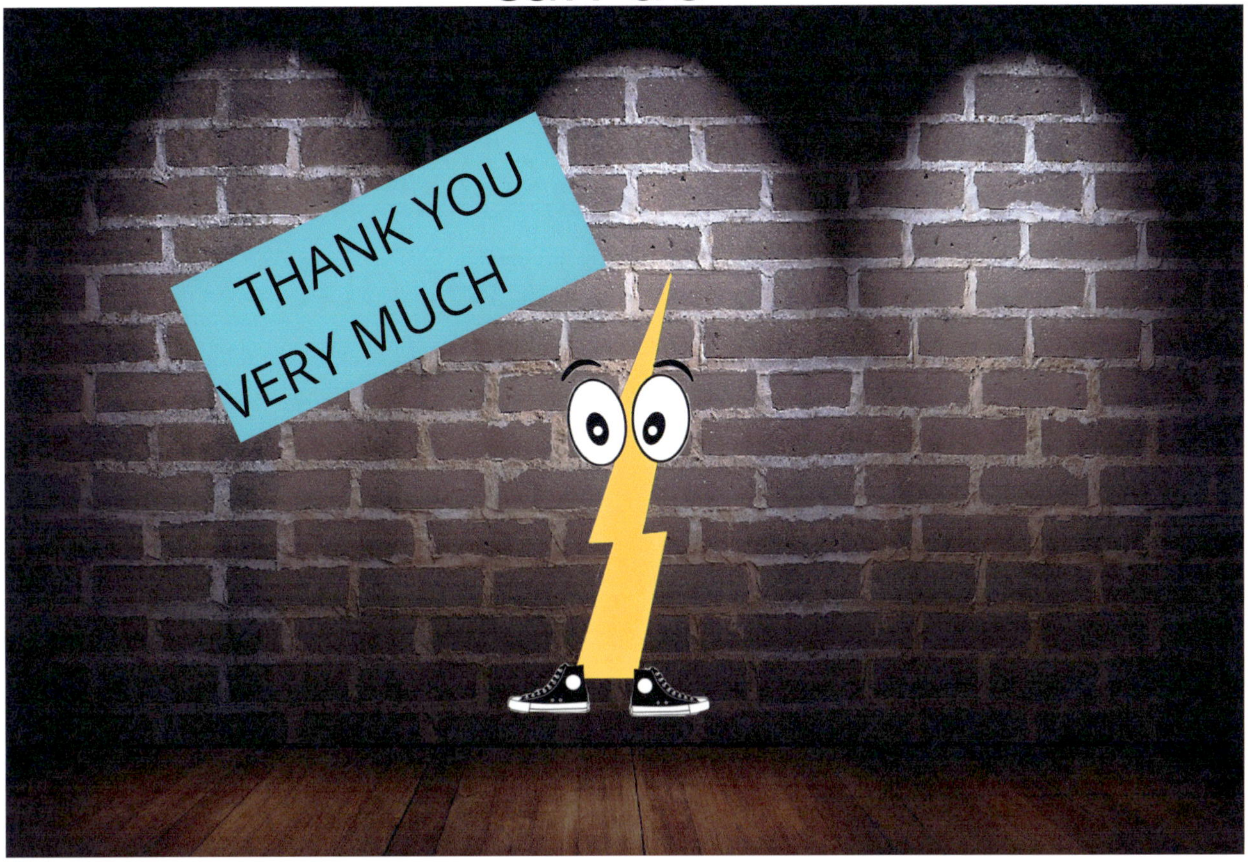

Polly is going to tell you a little about herself!

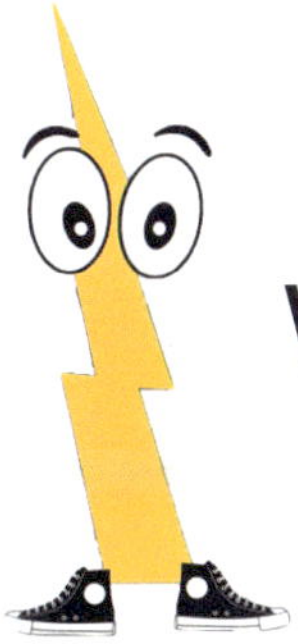

Wait!!! You are not Polly!!!

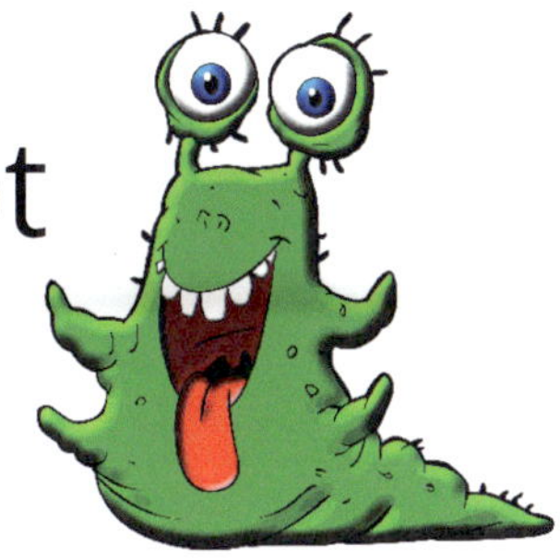

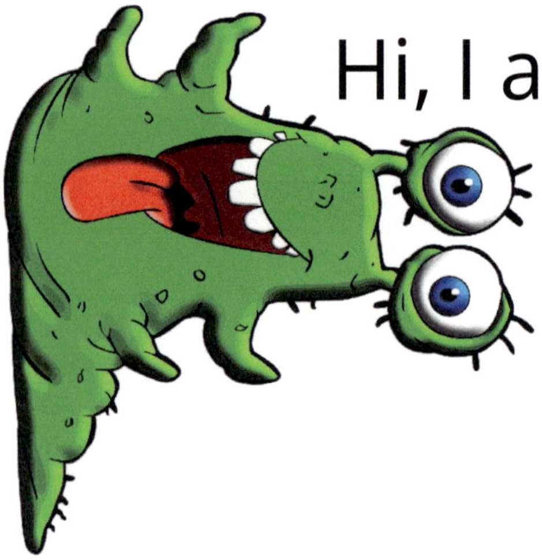

Hi, I am Polly!

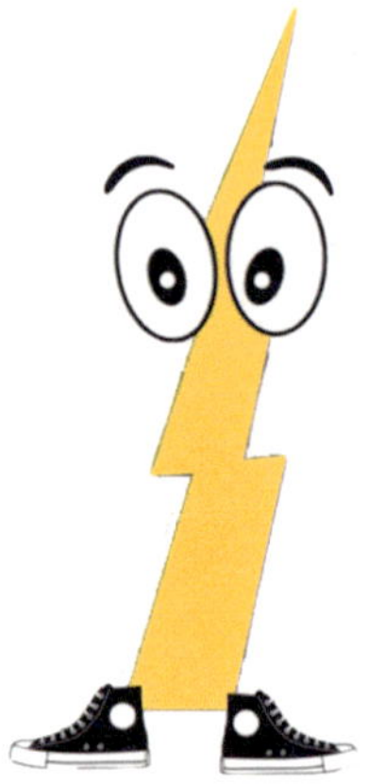

NO you are not!! Get out of here!!

COULD SOMEONE GET ARLEEN OUT OF HERE???!!

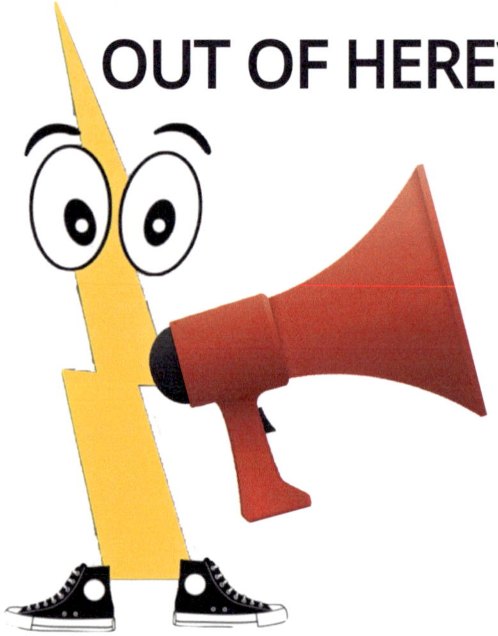

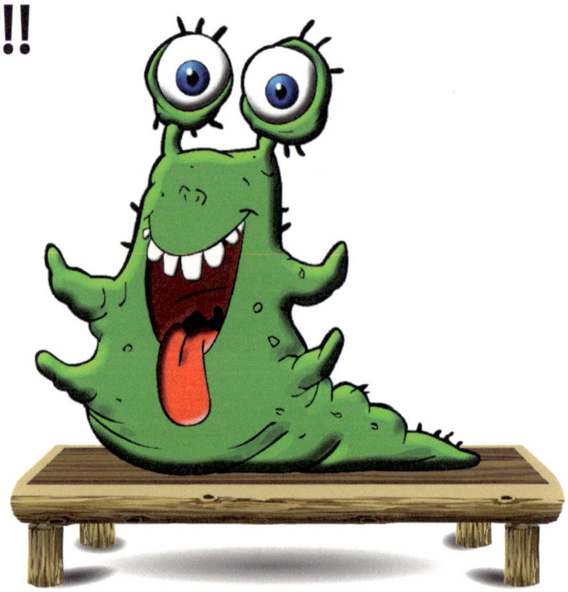

WHERE IS POLLY???

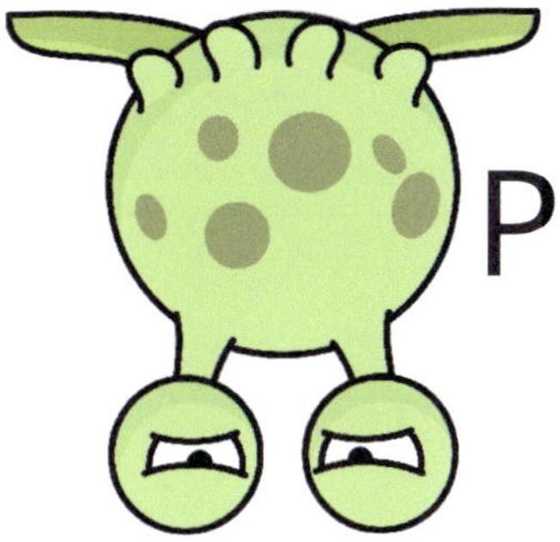

POLLY???

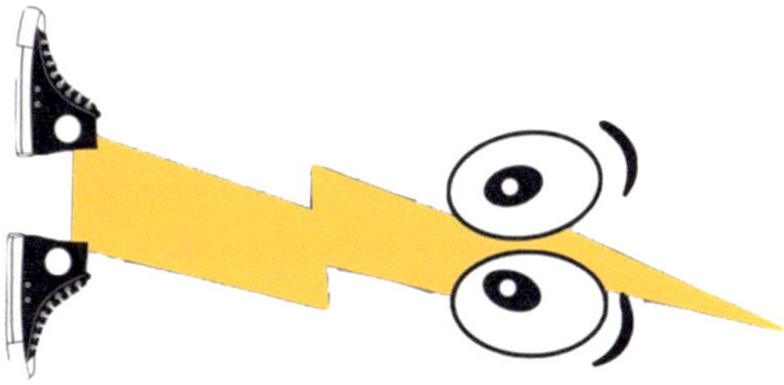

POLLY??? WHERE ARE YOU??

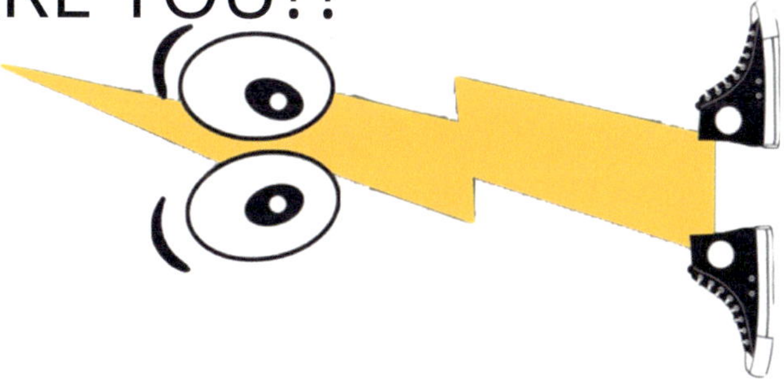

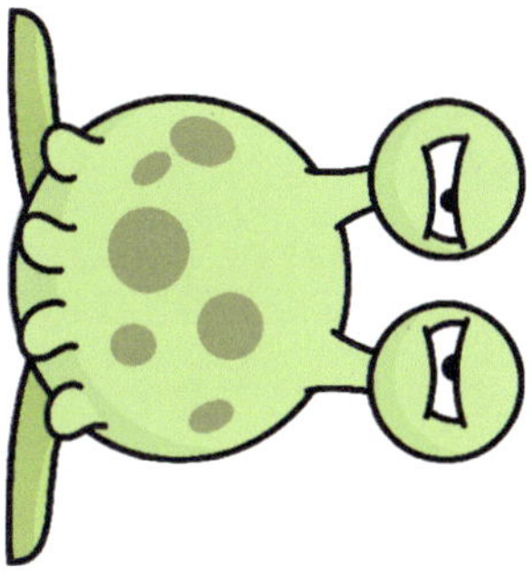

POLLY!!!!!!!!!!!

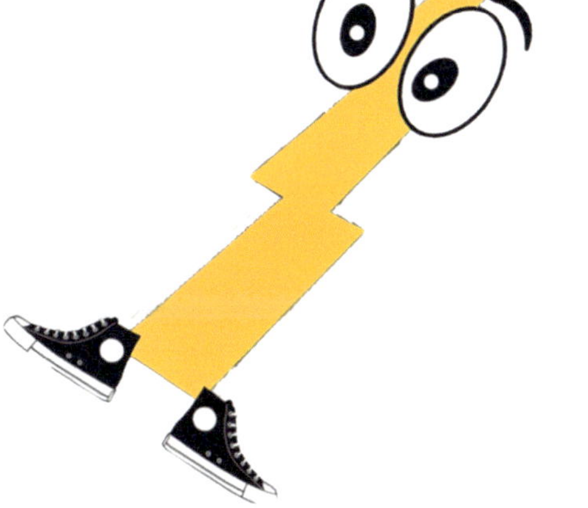

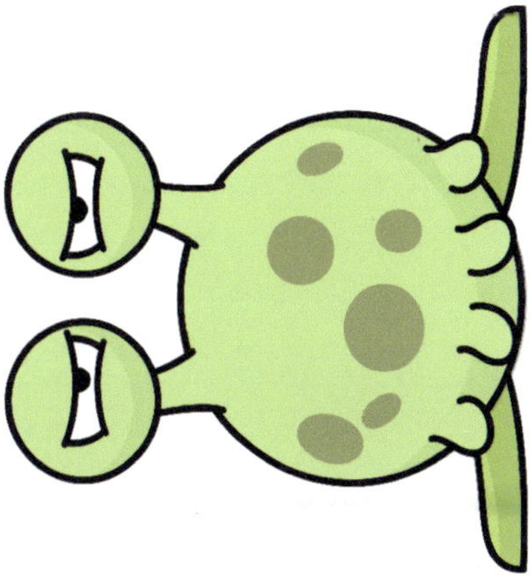

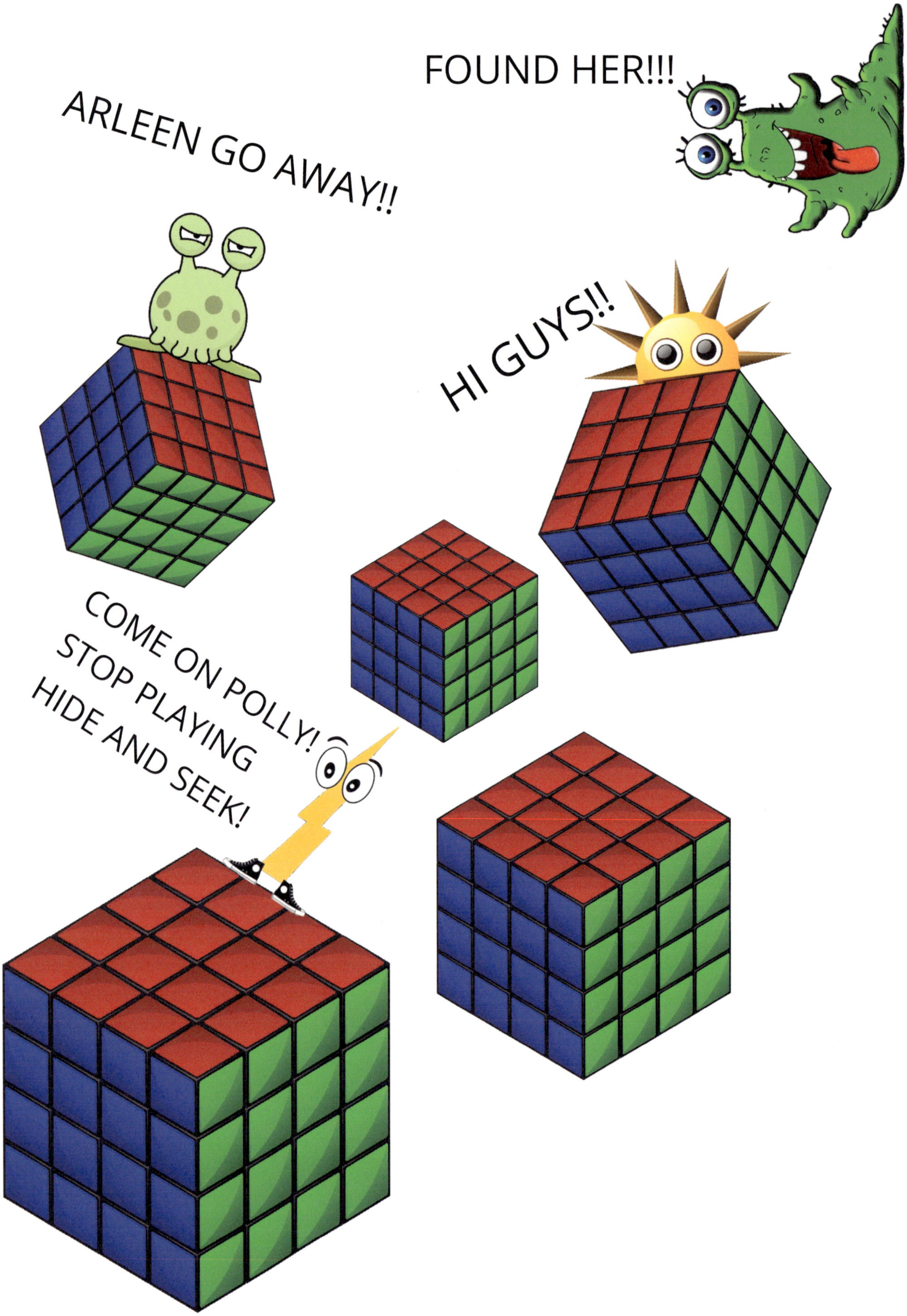
FOUND HER!!!
ARLEEN GO AWAY!!
HI GUYS!!
COME ON POLLY!
STOP PLAYING
HIDE AND SEEK!

Polly, enough hide and seek!! Time to tell the people all about yourself!

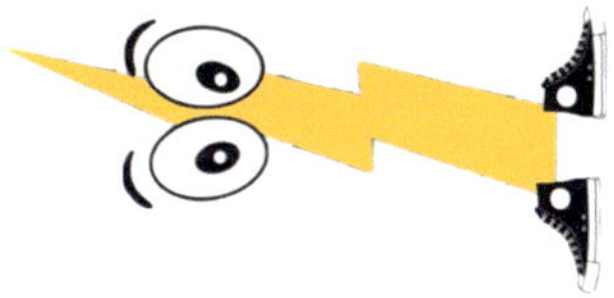

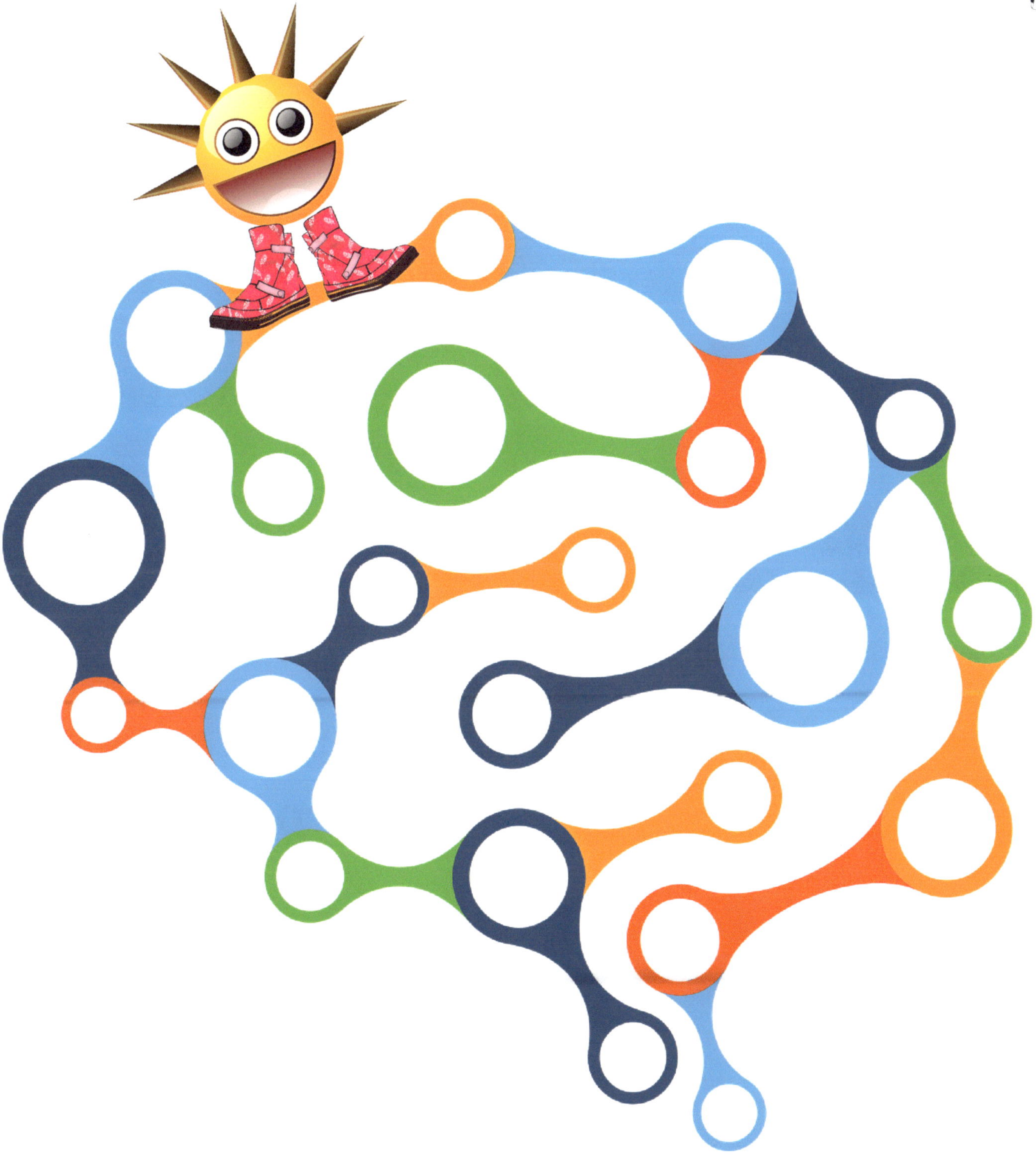

As you have heard, my name is Polly. My real name is Polly Spike. I am Spike's cousin.

He will not tell you this, but I am faster than he is!

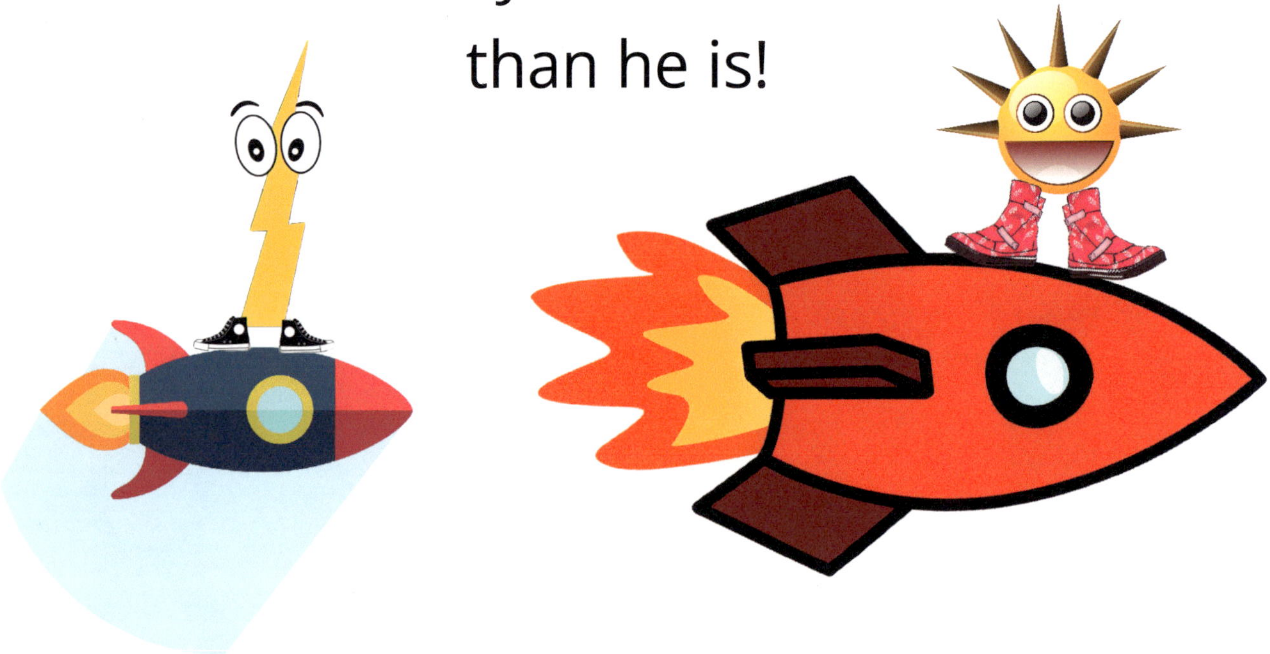

I can make electrical spikes much faster than my cousin! Let me show you...

I can cause seizures just like my cousin. I can make the electrical spikes really tall and strong if I want to. I make more than 1 spike happen at a time.

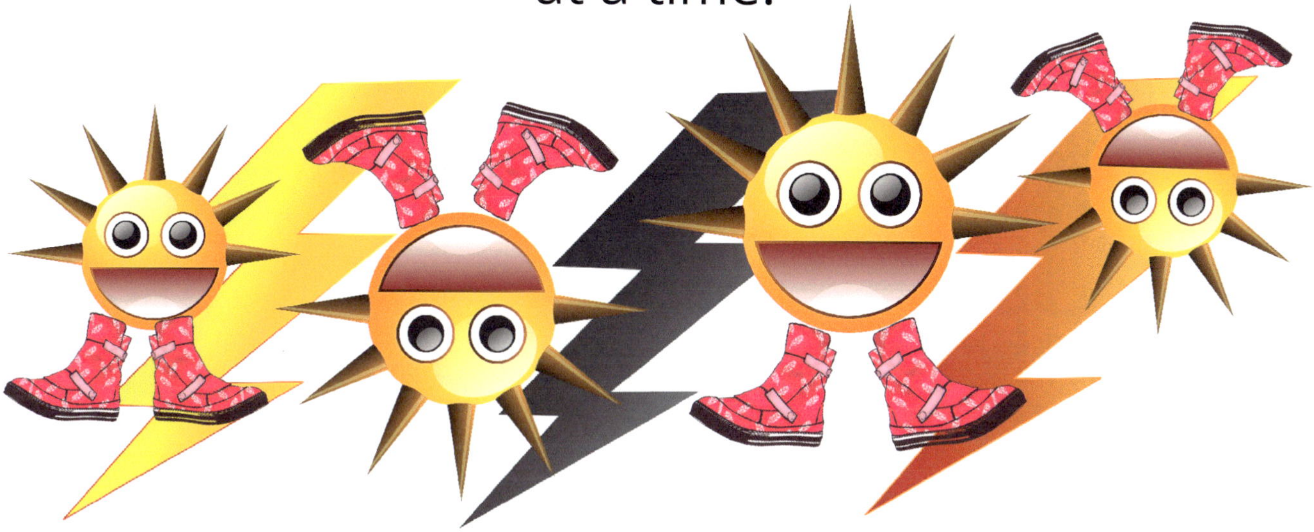

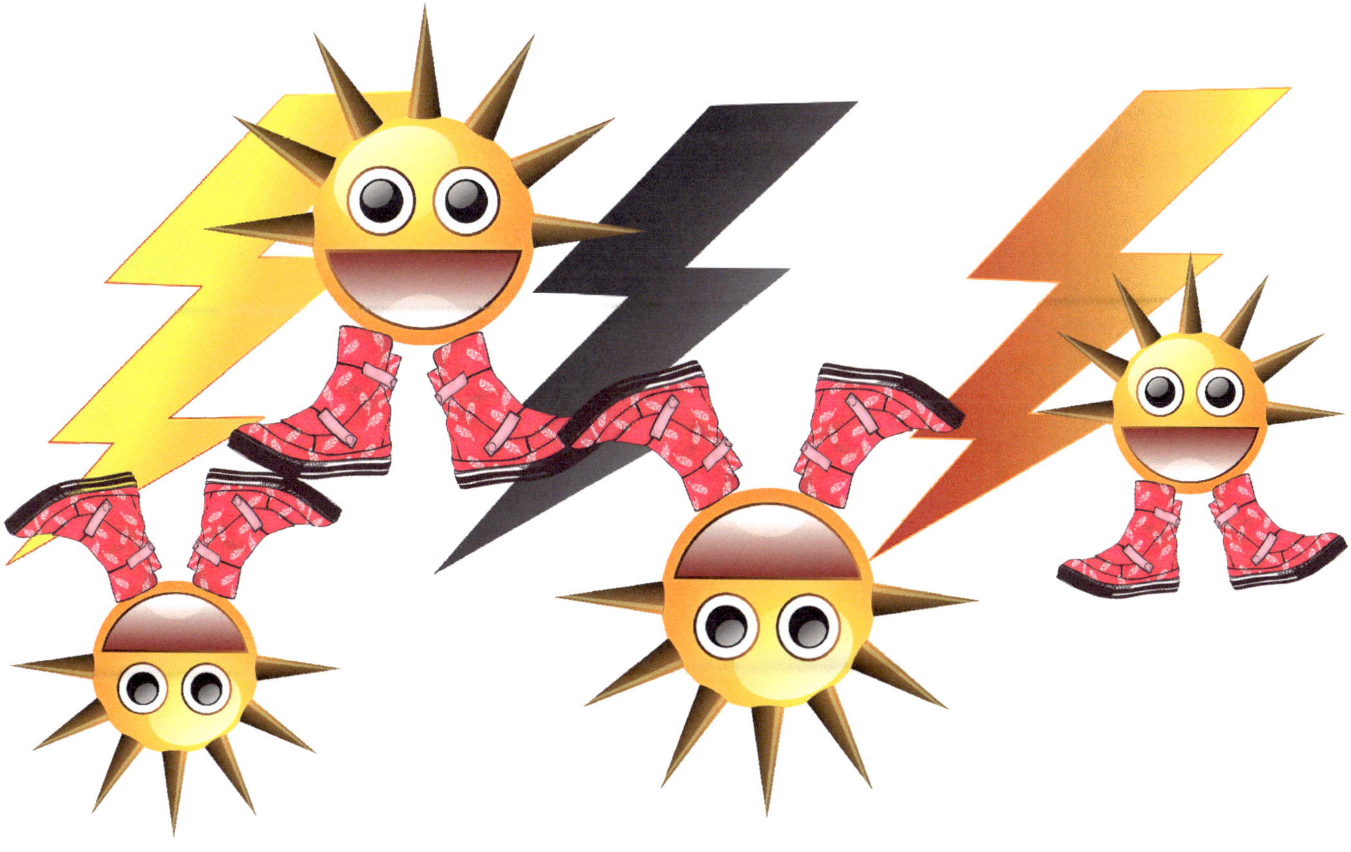

Sometimes Spike and I make trouble together! We love it but no one else does!

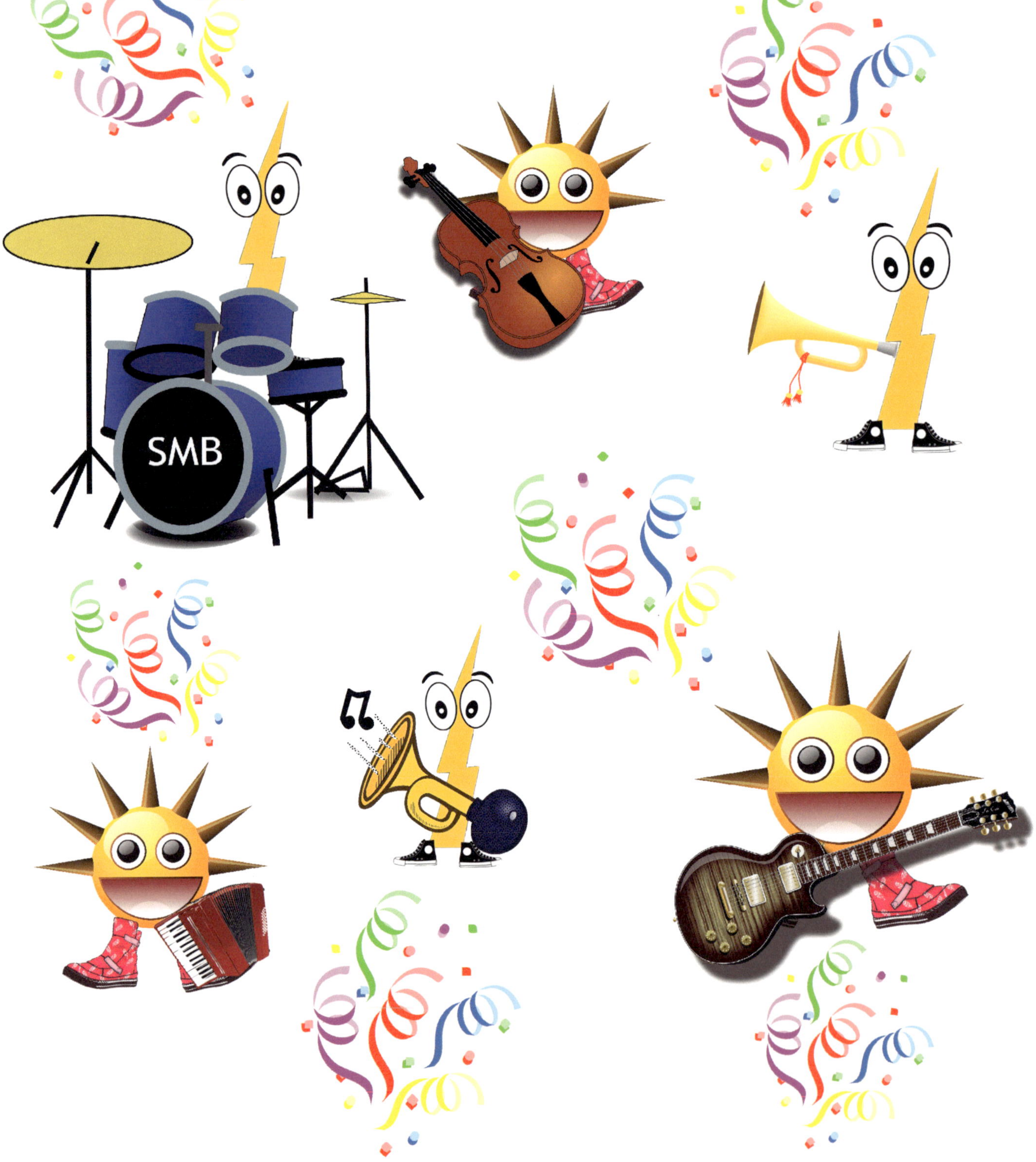

Now you know what I can do and

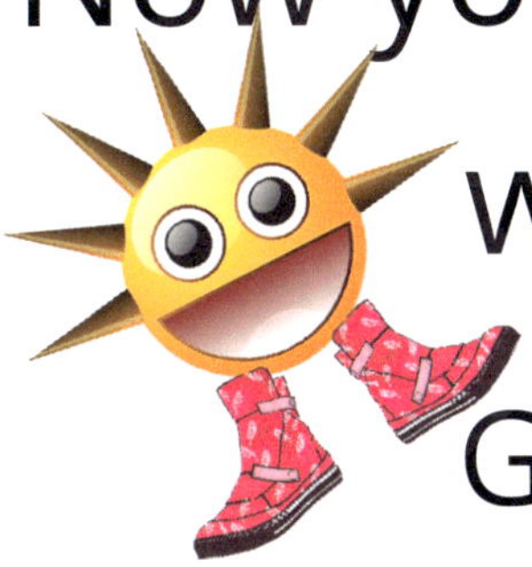

why no one likes us.

Guess I will go play now,

so let me turn it back

over to Spike!

SPIKE!!

SPIKE!!??

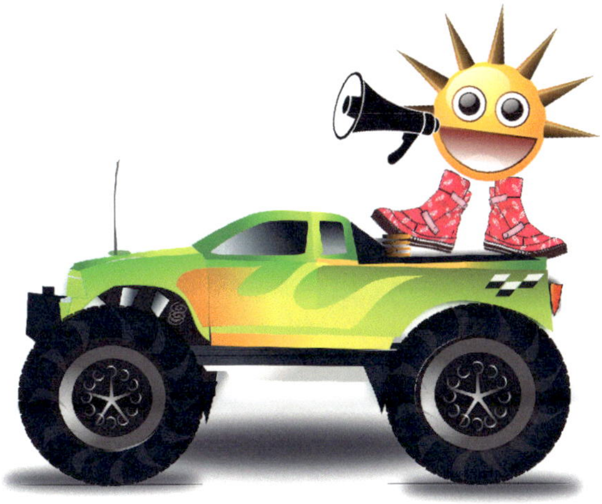

Hi there! I am Freddy Frontal!

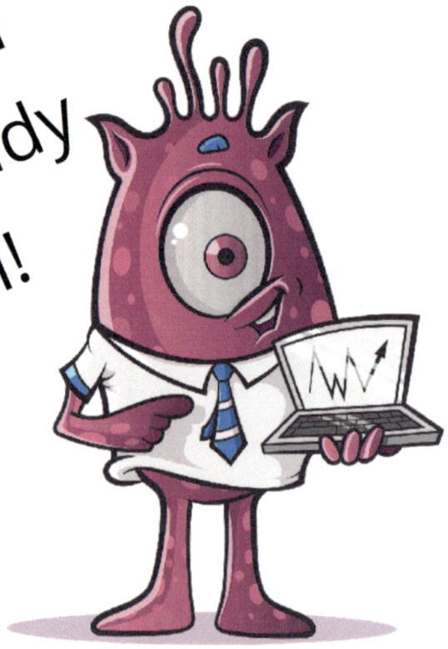

Freddy, you showed up on the wrong day!! You are not in this book!!

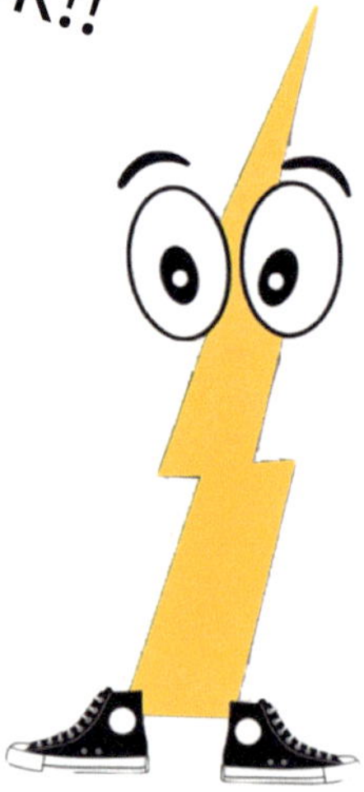

And someone get Arleen out of here!!!

Sharpie, it is your turn!

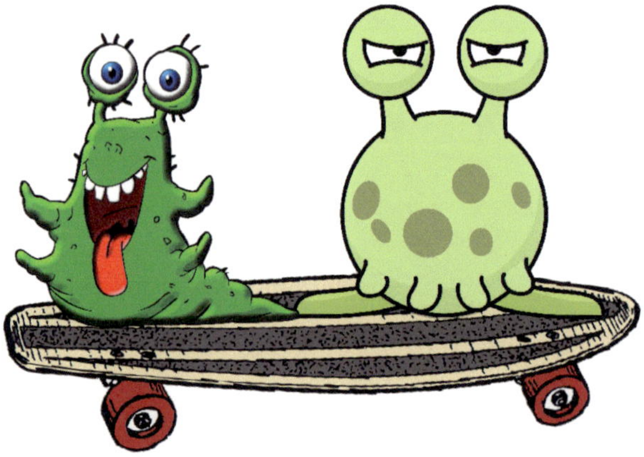

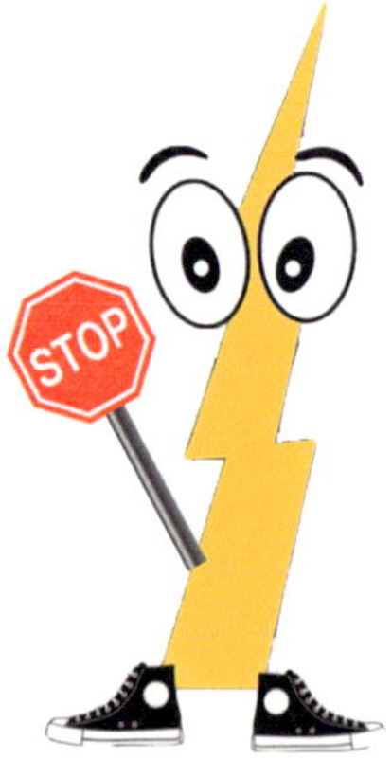

My name is Sharpie. I am not as strong as Spike and Polly, but I still know how to start trouble. I usually like to sit back and let those two do the hard work.

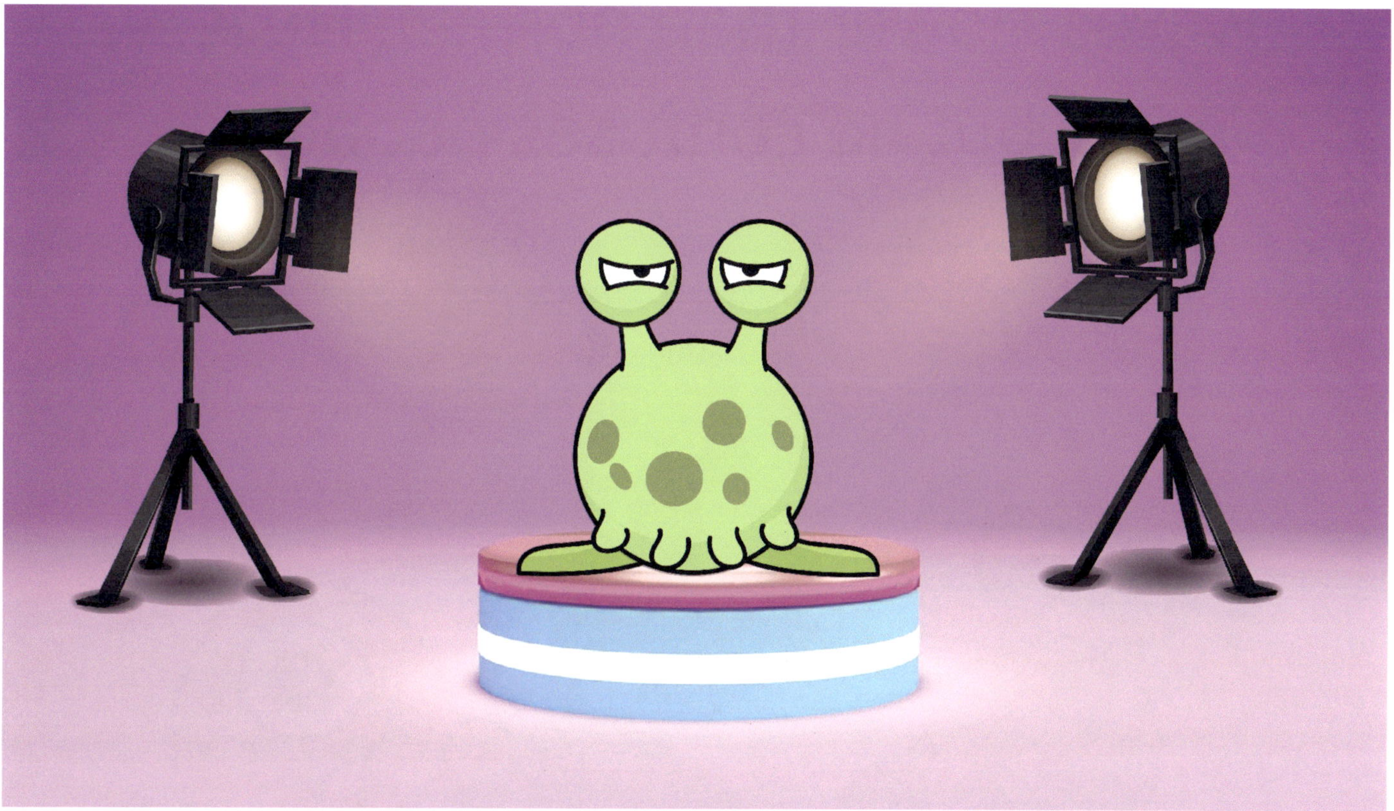

I can hide out anywhere in your brain when I want to. Sometimes I hang out alone.

Sometimes I hang out with my friend Slowpoke. He makes brain waves slower than normal. He is nice, but he confuses people.

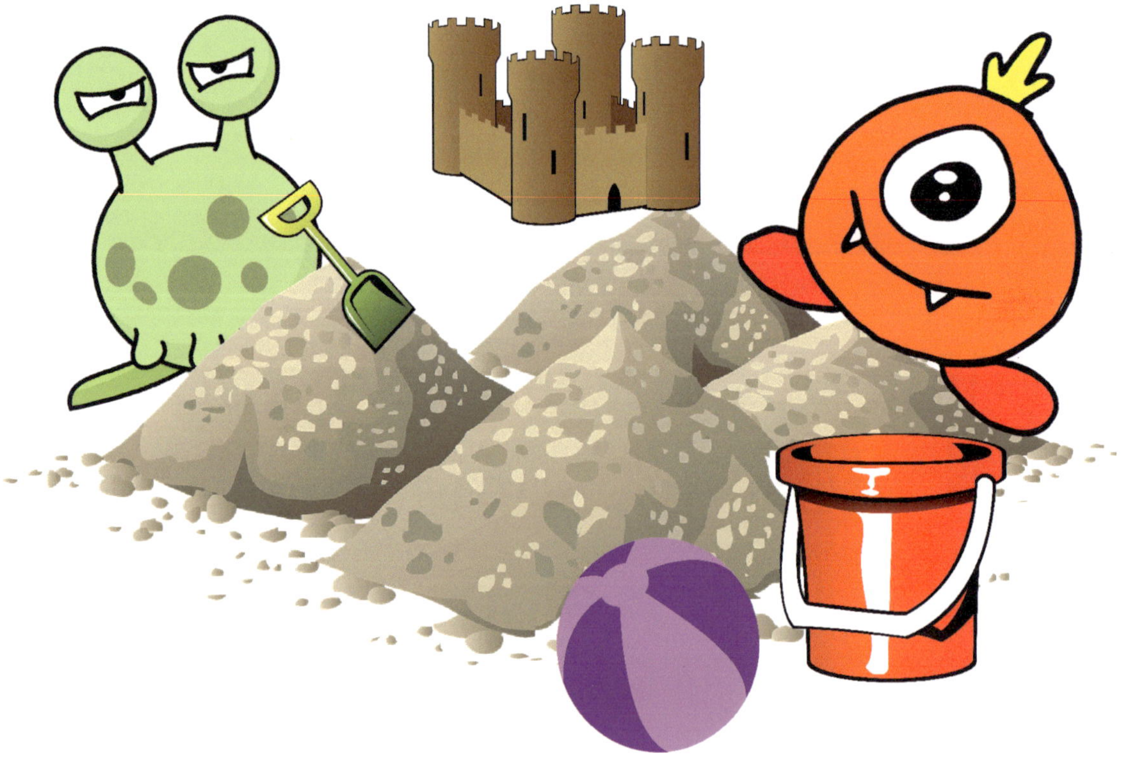

We can make a real mess when we all hang out together

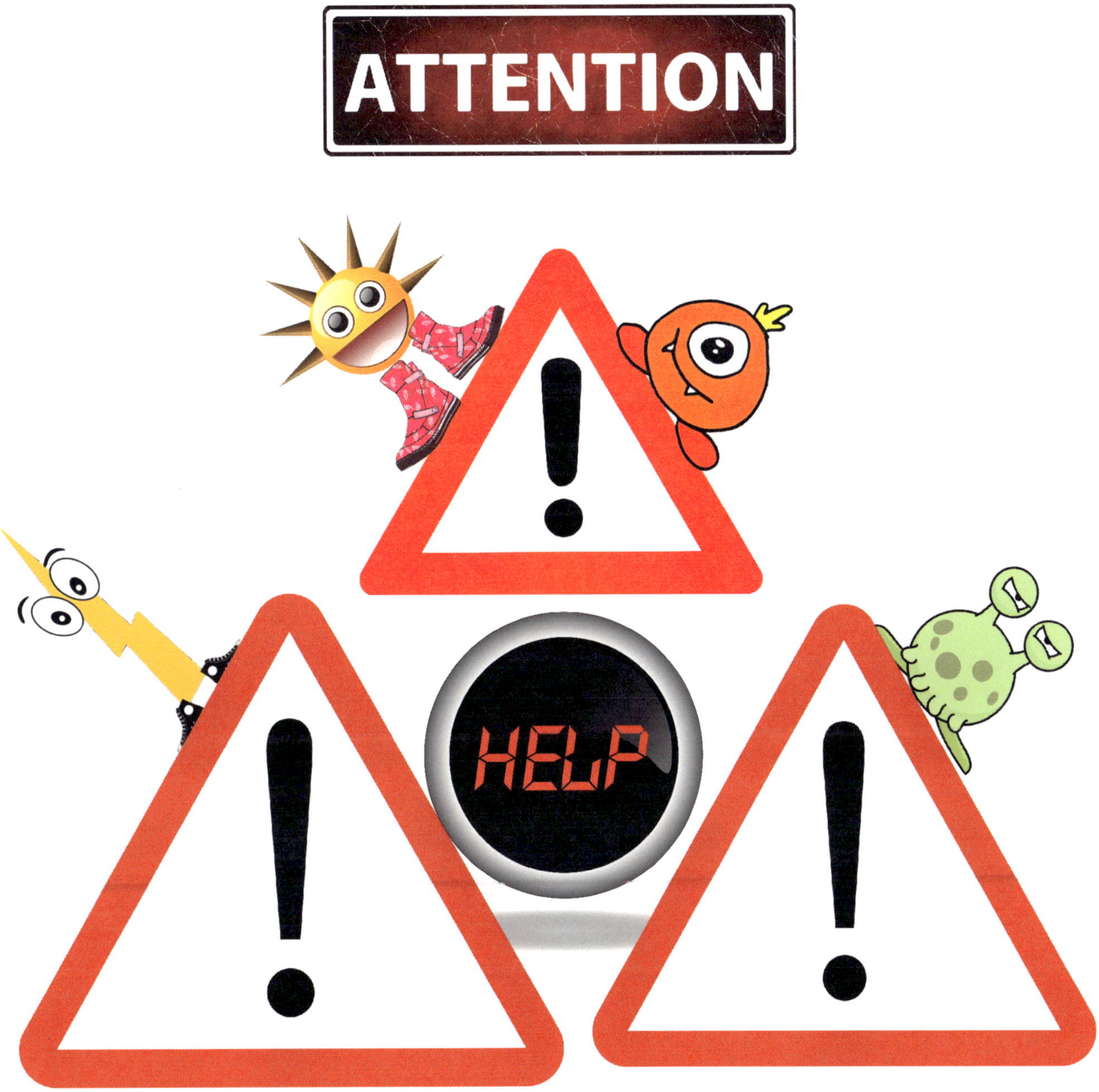

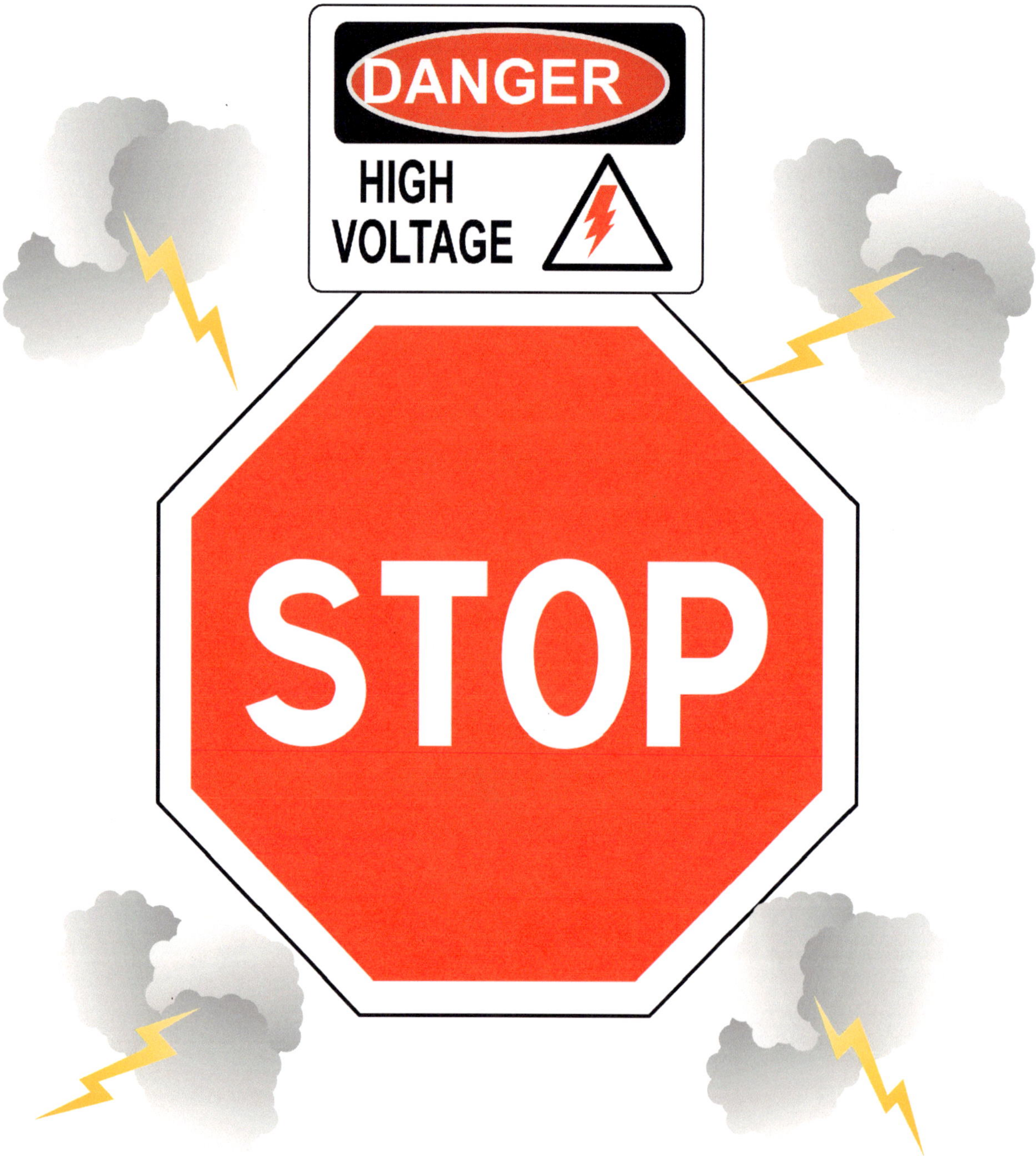
DANGER
HIGH
VOLTAGE
STOP

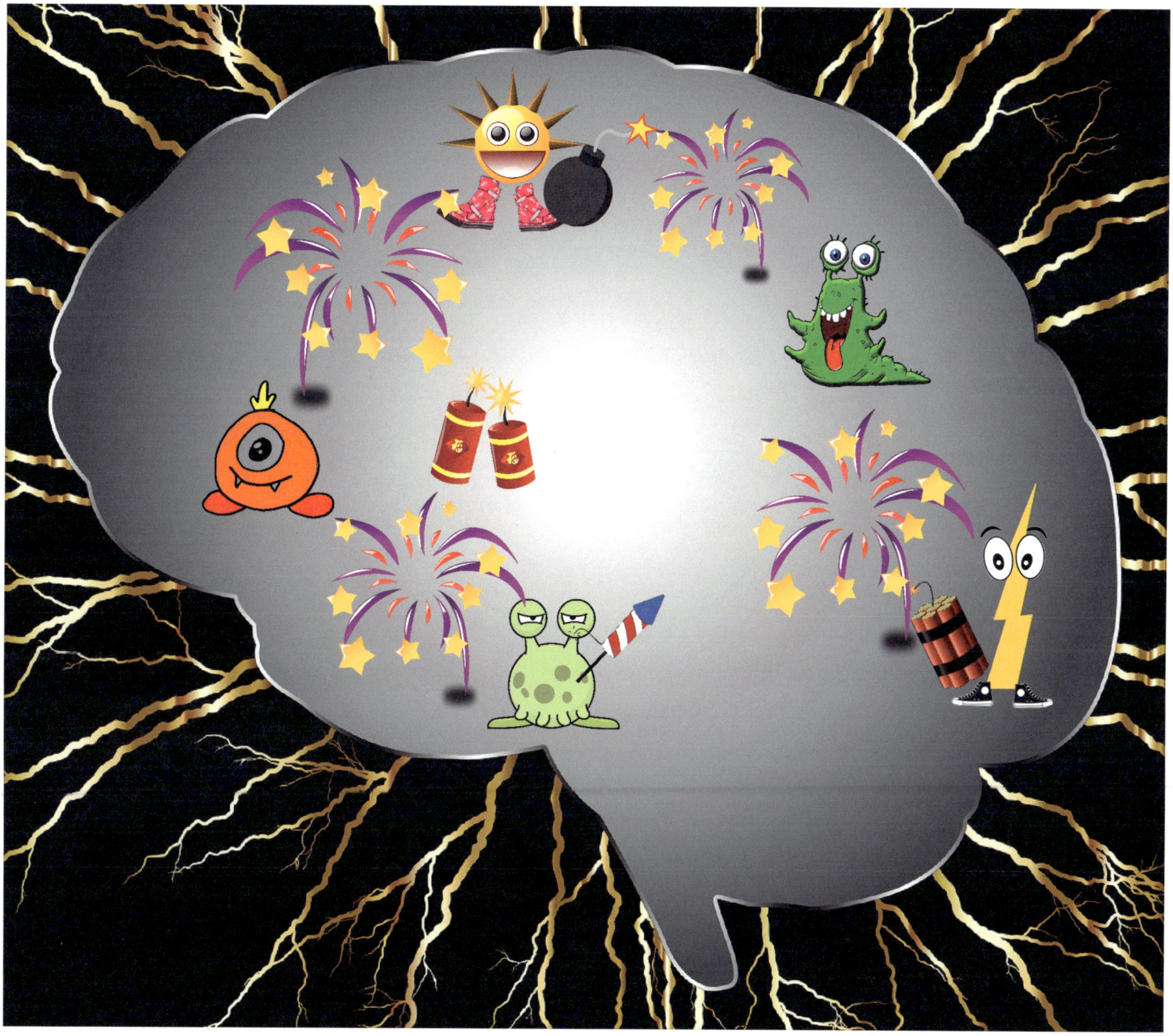

Arleen, get out of here!!!!

I am Arleen Artifact (are-tee-fact)!! I am important!!

I got her! Come on Arleen, time to go!!

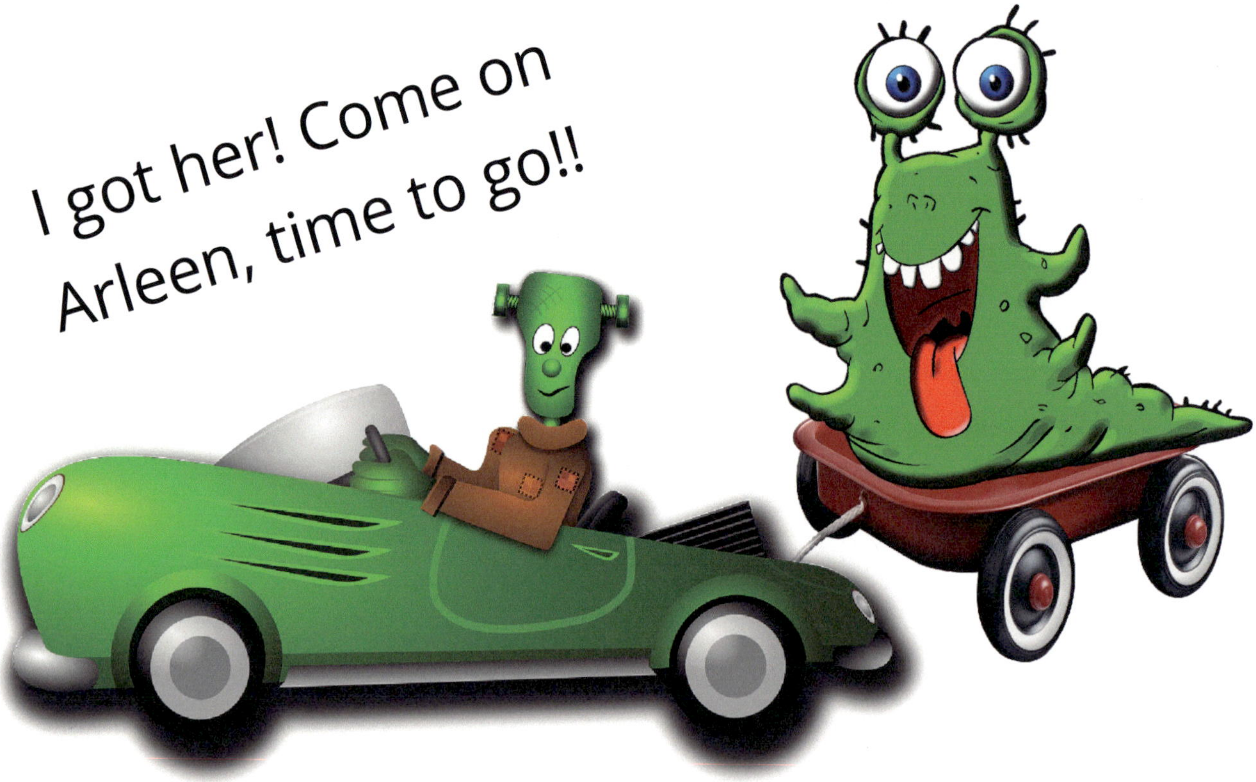

It is not your turn Arleen!! See you later! We will call you!

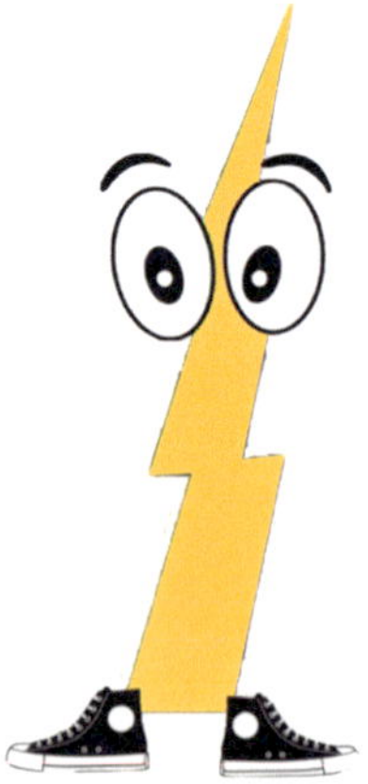

Well, now you know a little about each of us. We can work alone or together.

We do not mean to cause trouble, but we can't help it. Trouble is fun!!

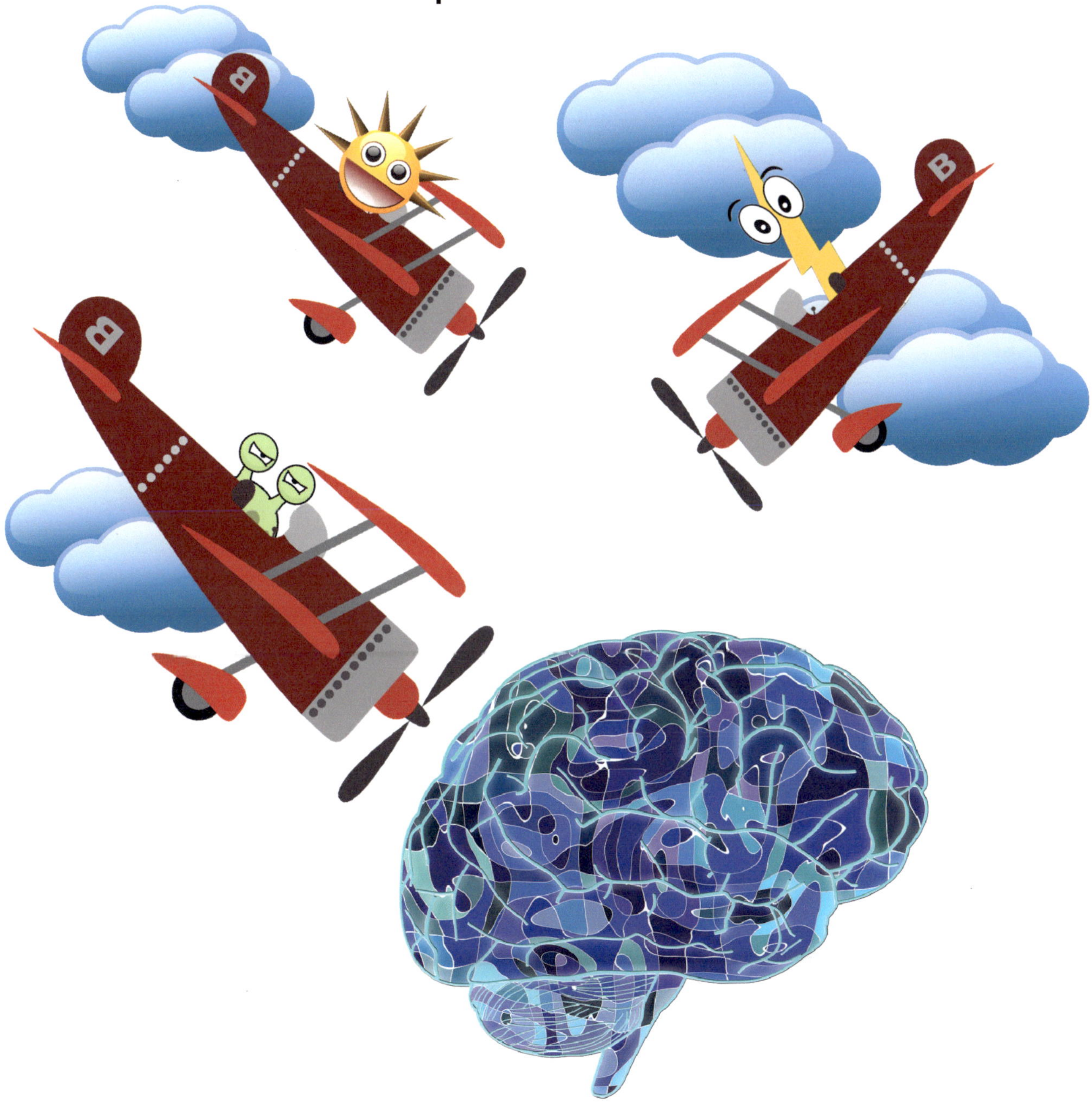

So now you know a little bit more about seizures.

We talked about what we can do and what it does to you and your brain.

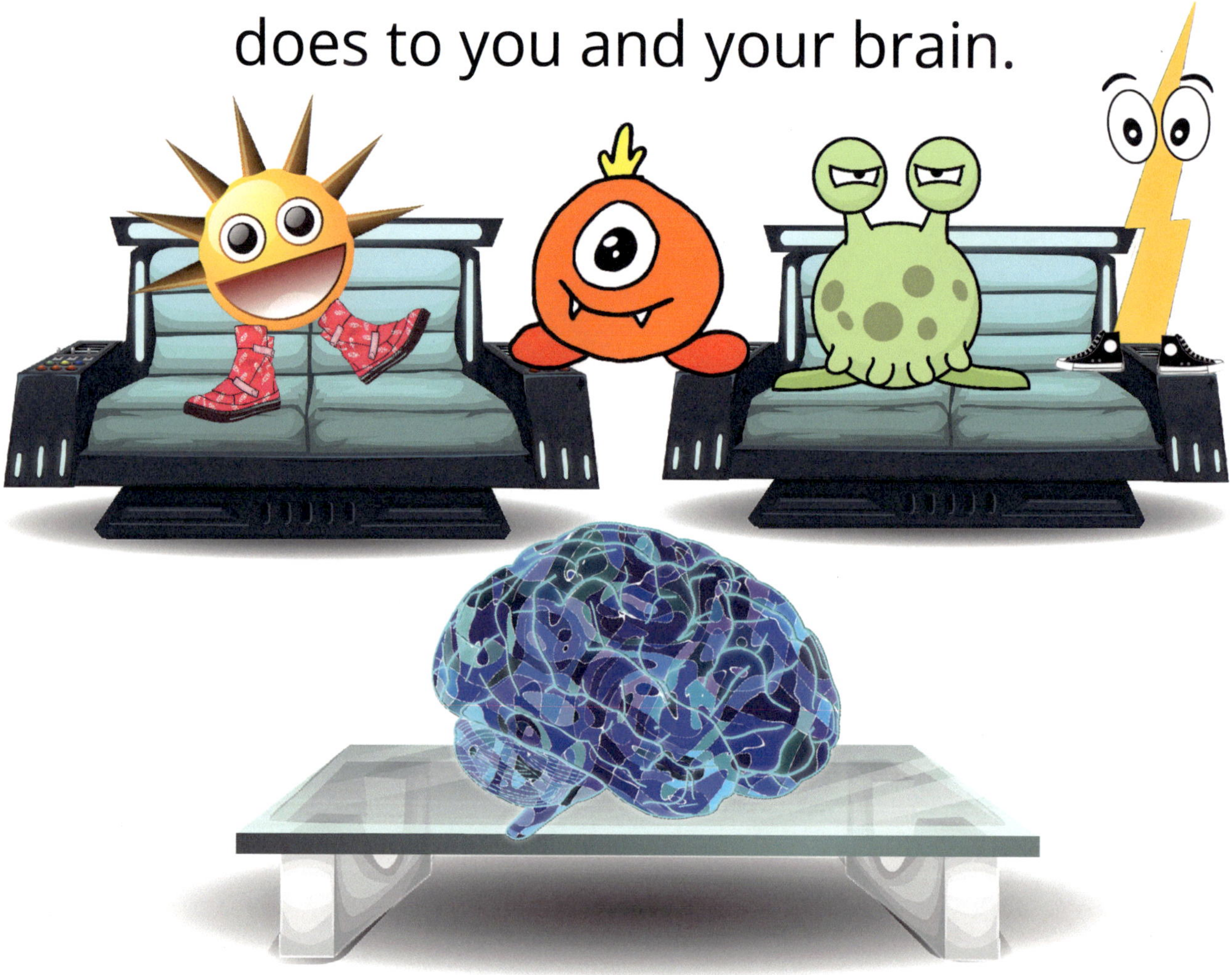

We should let you get some rest as we have been talking a lot.

We are ready to enjoy a relaxing evening.

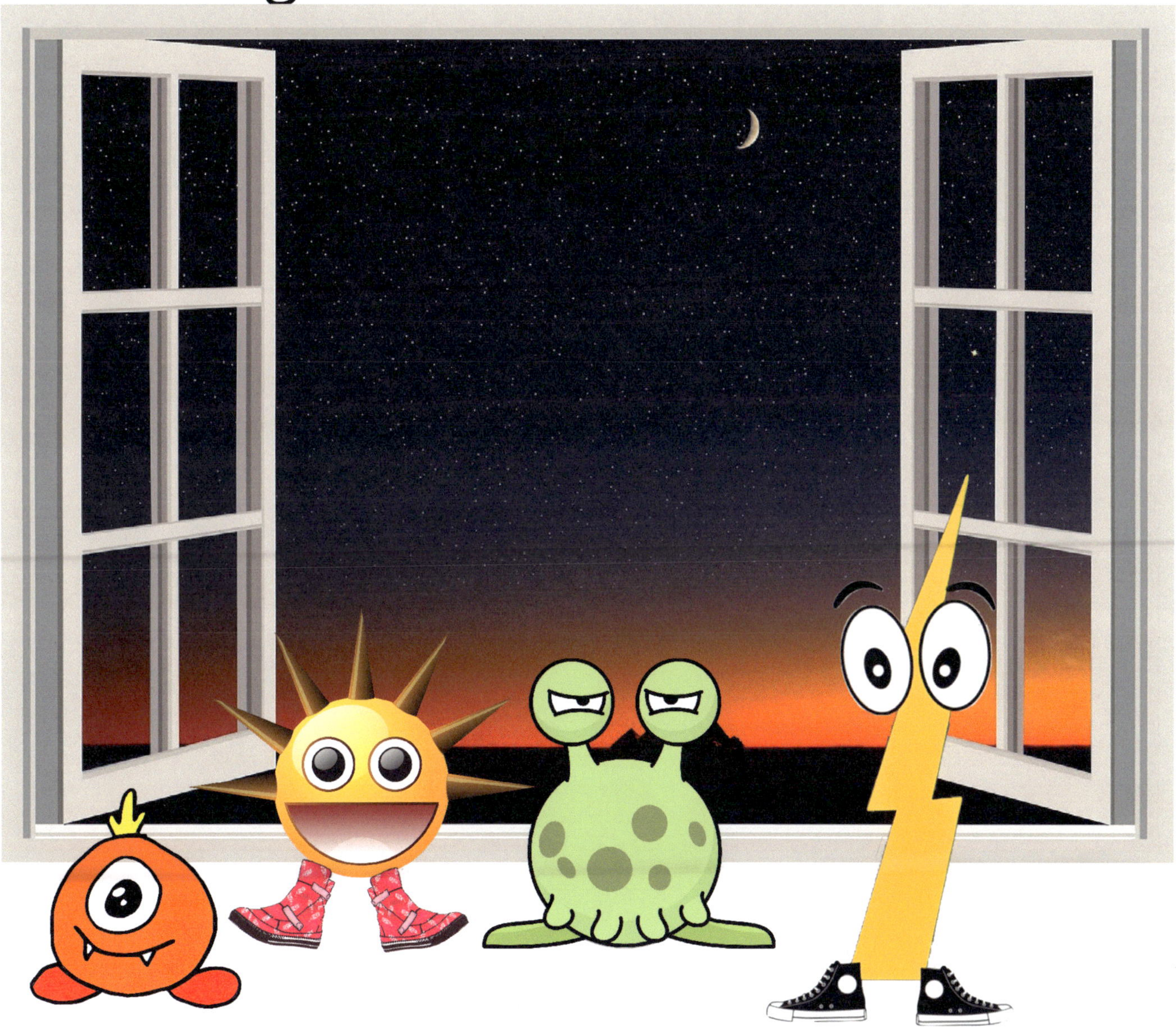

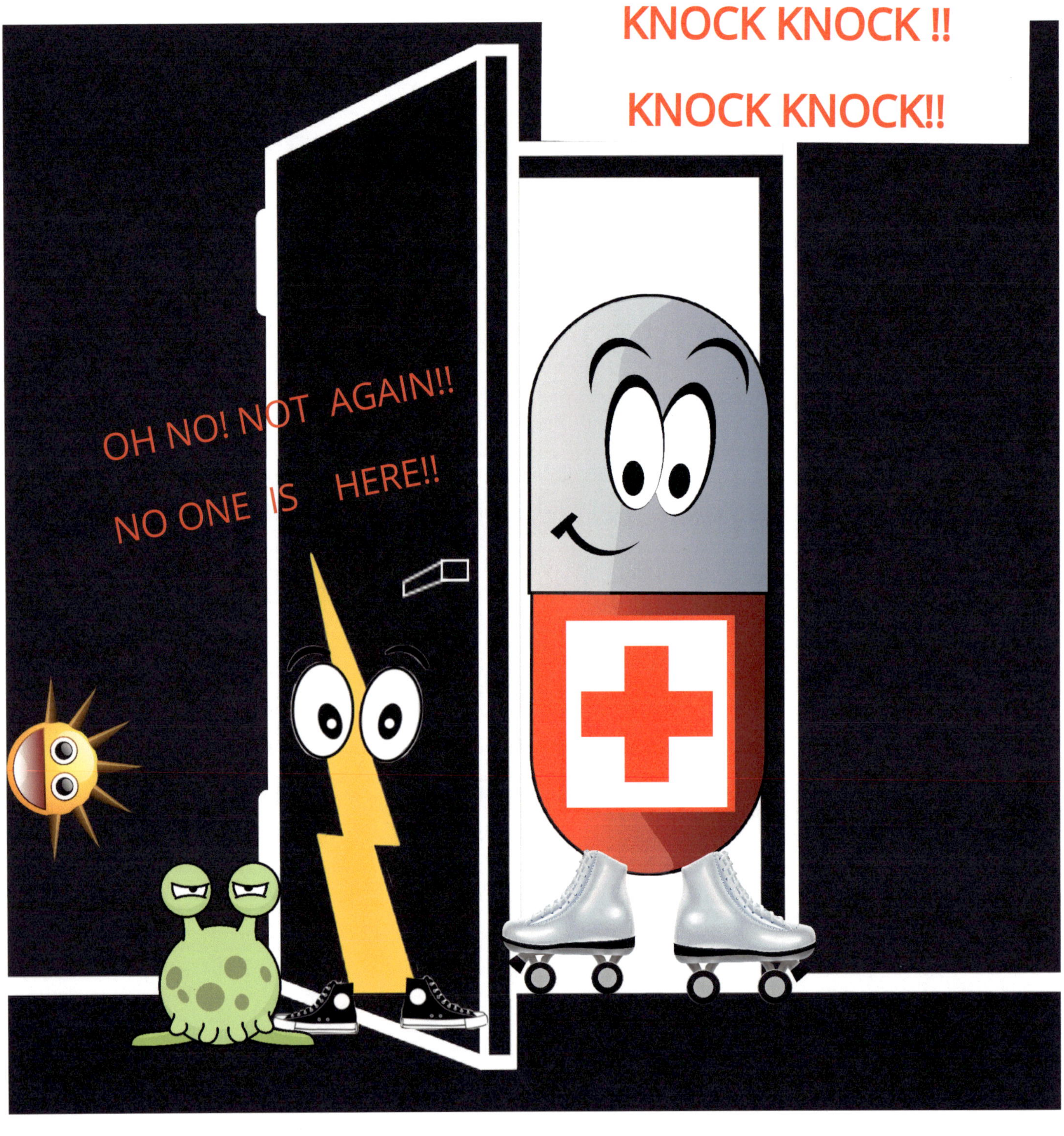
KNOCK KNOCK !!
KNOCK KNOCK!!
OH NO! NOT AGAIN!!
NO ONE IS HERE!!

Time for you and your gang to move on. We have taken over this part of the brain. You are not welcome!

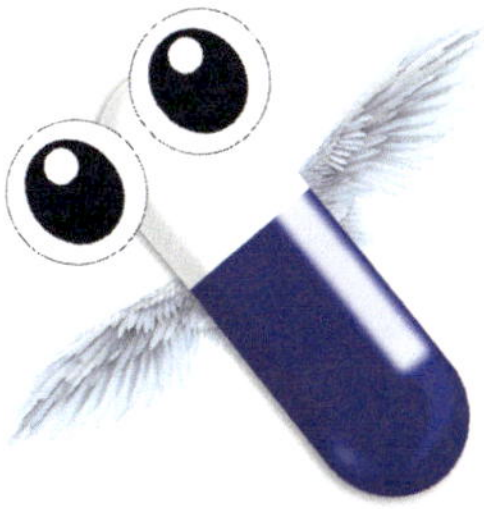

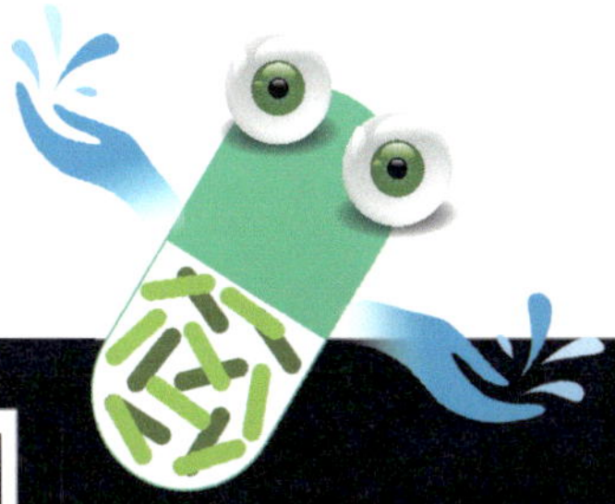

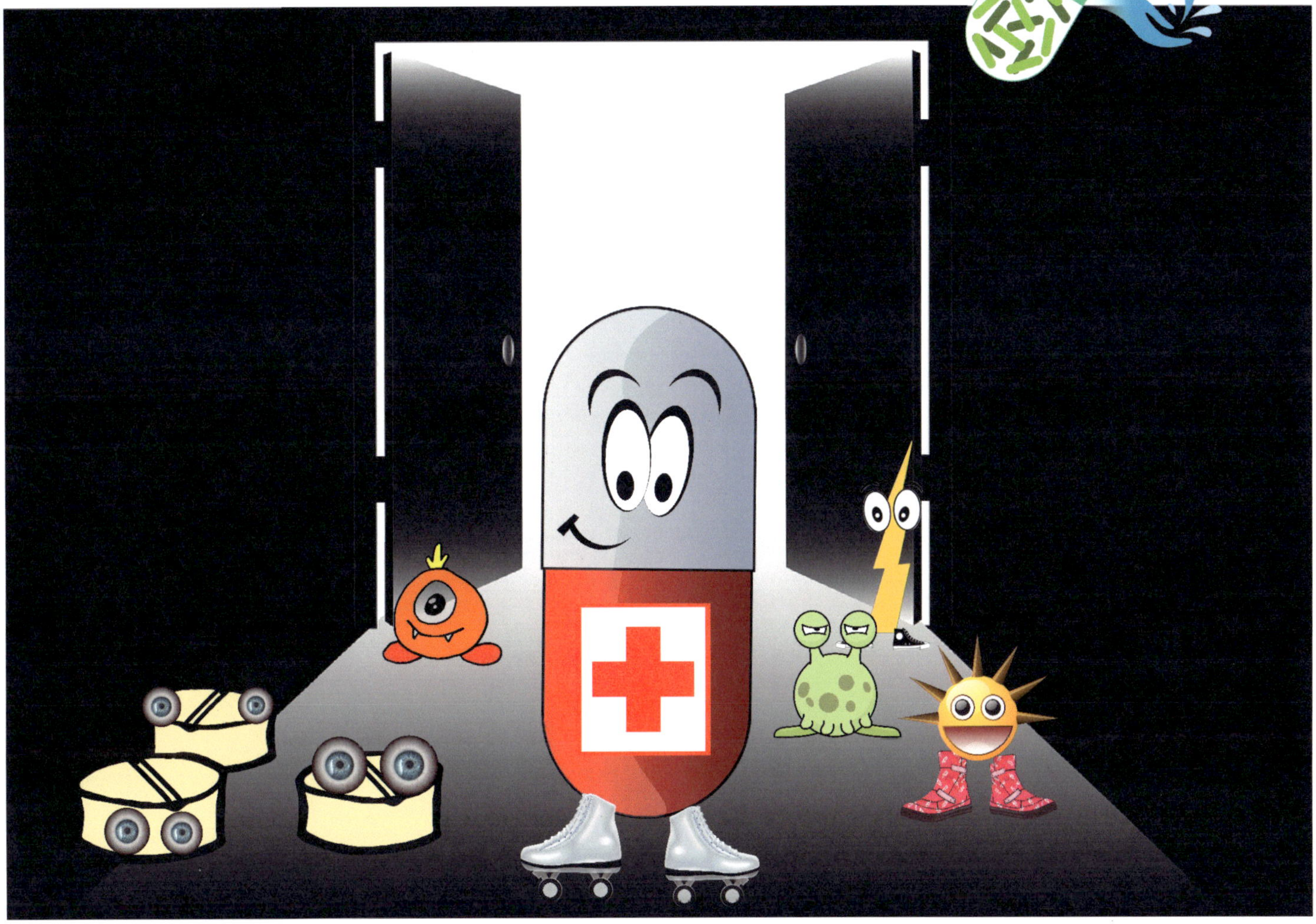

Brain protected by Super Med and the Crew

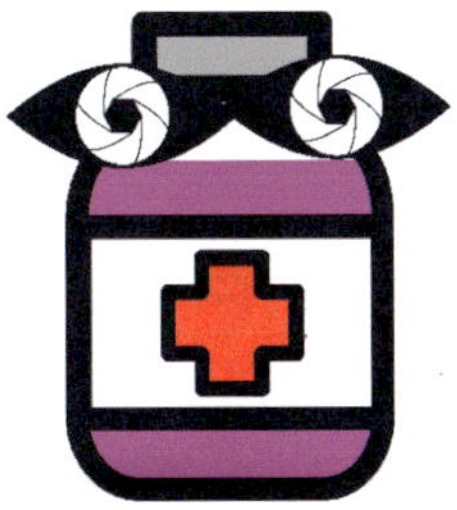

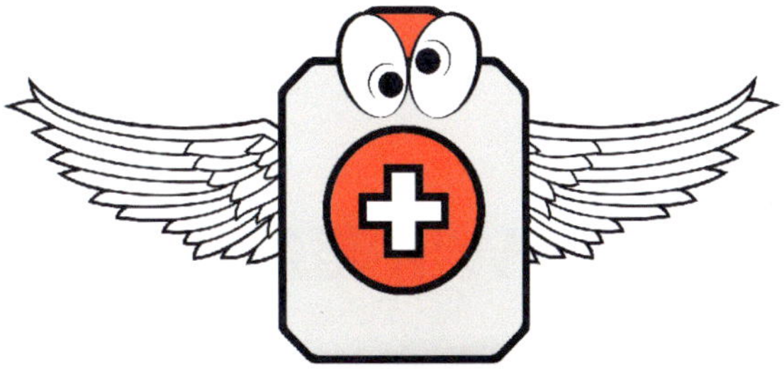

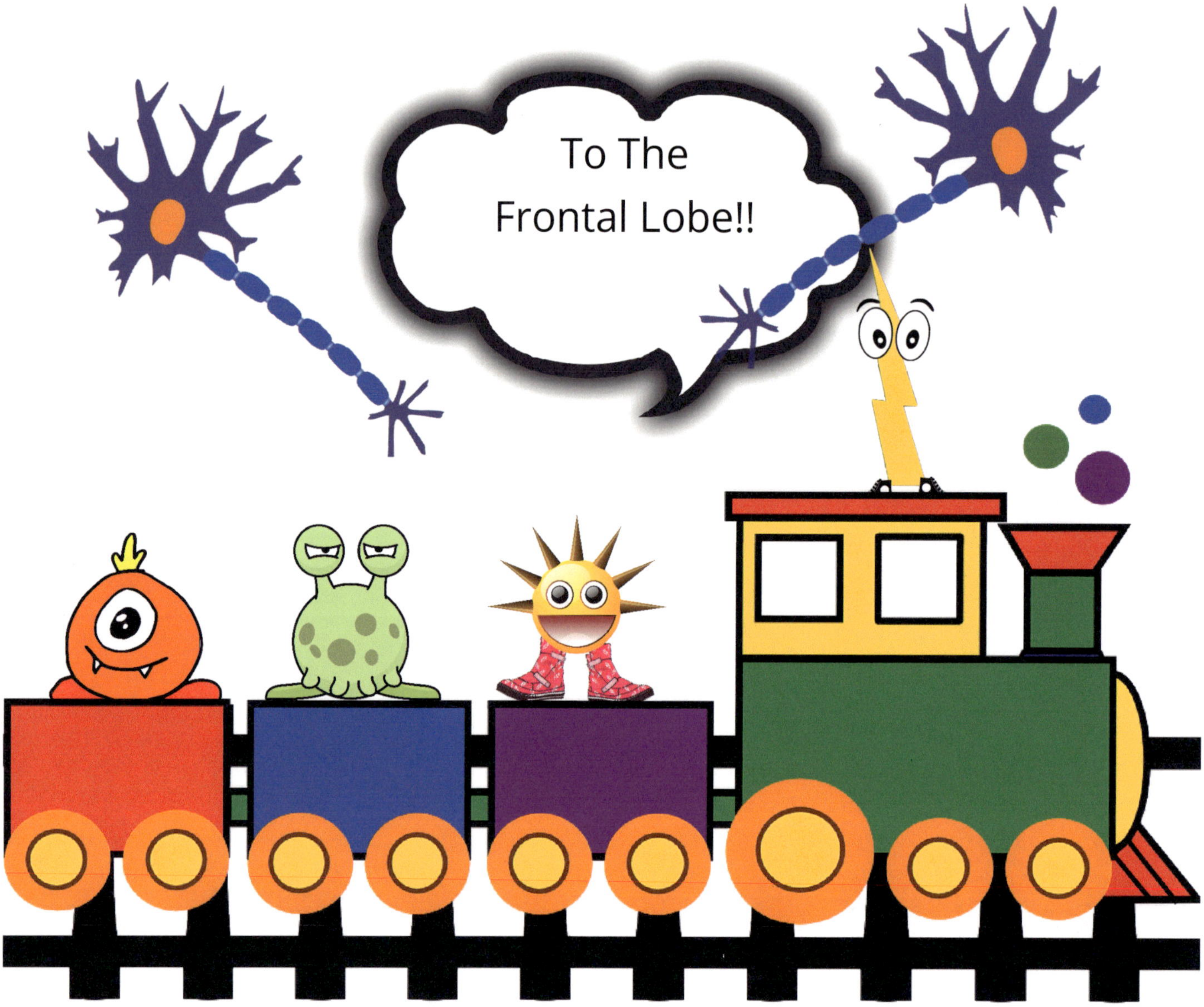

Don't tell Super Med and the Crew where we are going!! It's a secret!!

We will be back to cause more trouble soon!!

SEE YOU SOON!!!

THE GANG WILL BE BACK SOON!!!

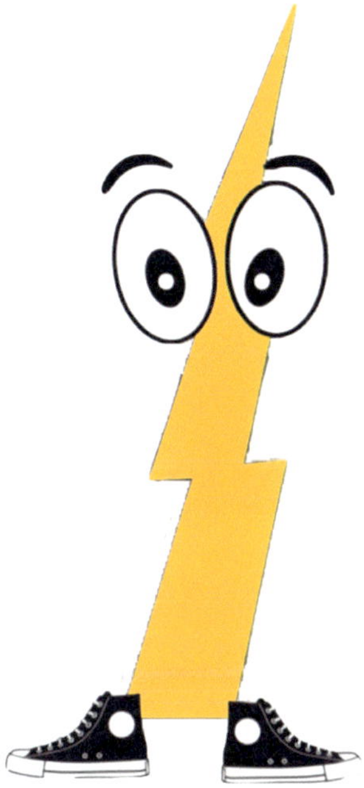

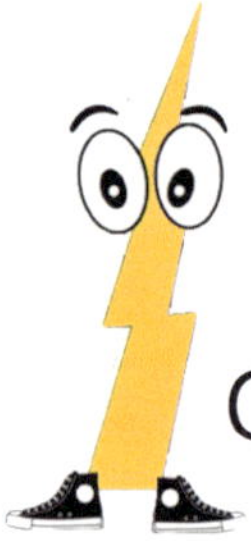

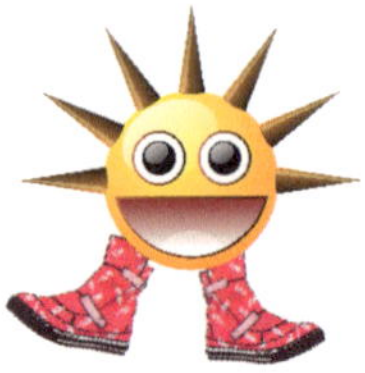

Stay tuned for The Gang Meets Freddy Frontal

Book 3: Coming early 2022!

Find all the Books in the Let's Learn About Epilepsy Series at

www.spikeandthegang.com and major retailers

Follow Spike and the Gang on Instagram, Twitter

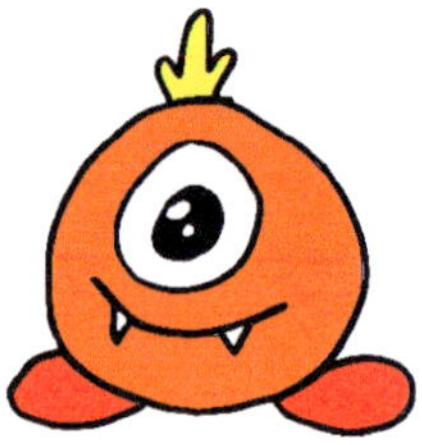

and Facebook

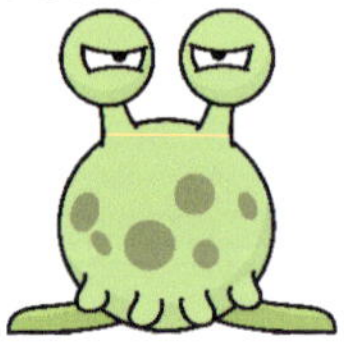

And would someone get Arlene out of here!!!

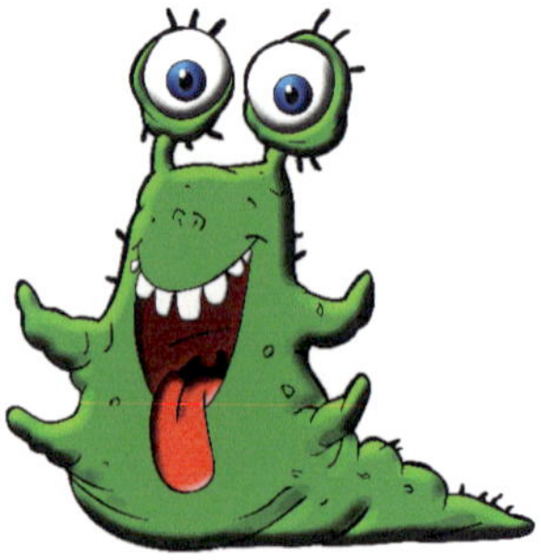

Made in the USA
Las Vegas, NV
07 November 2026

57673306R00024